Dental Communication

David W. Chambers, Ed.M., M.B.A., Ph.D.
Professor and Director, Division of
Educational Development and Management
School of Dentistry, University of the Pacific
San Francisco, California

Ronald G. Abrams, D.M.D., M.S.
Professor of Pediatric Dentistry
Baltimore College of Dental Surgery
University of Maryland Dental School
Baltimore, Maryland

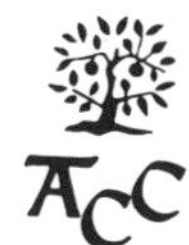

APPLETON-CENTURY-CROFTS/Norwalk, Connecticut

0-8385-1572-X

Notice: The author(s) and publisher of this volume have taken care that the information and recommendations contained herein are accurate and compatible with the standards generally accepted at the time of publication.

86 87 88 89 / 10 9 8 7 6 5 4 3 2 1

Prentice-Hall of Australia, Pty. Ltd., Sydney
Prentice-Hall Canada, Inc.
Prentice-Hall Hispanoamericana, S.A., Mexico
Prentice-Hall of India Private Limited, New Delhi
Prentice-Hall International (UK) Limited, London
Prentice-Hall of Japan, Inc., Tokyo
Prentice-Hall of Southeast Asia (Pte.) Ltd., Singapore
Whitehall Books Ltd., Wellington, New Zealand
Editora Prentice-Hall do Brasil Ltda., Rio de Janeiro

Library of Congress Cataloging-in-Publication Data

Chambers, David W.
Dental communication.

Includes index.
1. Dentistry—Practice. 2. Interpersonal communication. 3. Dental personnel and patient. I. Abrams, Ronald G.. II. Title. [DNLM: 1. Communication. 2. Dental Offices—organization & administration. 3. Dentist-Patient Relations. WU 61 C444d]
RK58.C44 1986 617.6'023 85-20165
ISBN 0-8385-1572-X

PRINTED IN THE UNITED STATES OF AMERICA

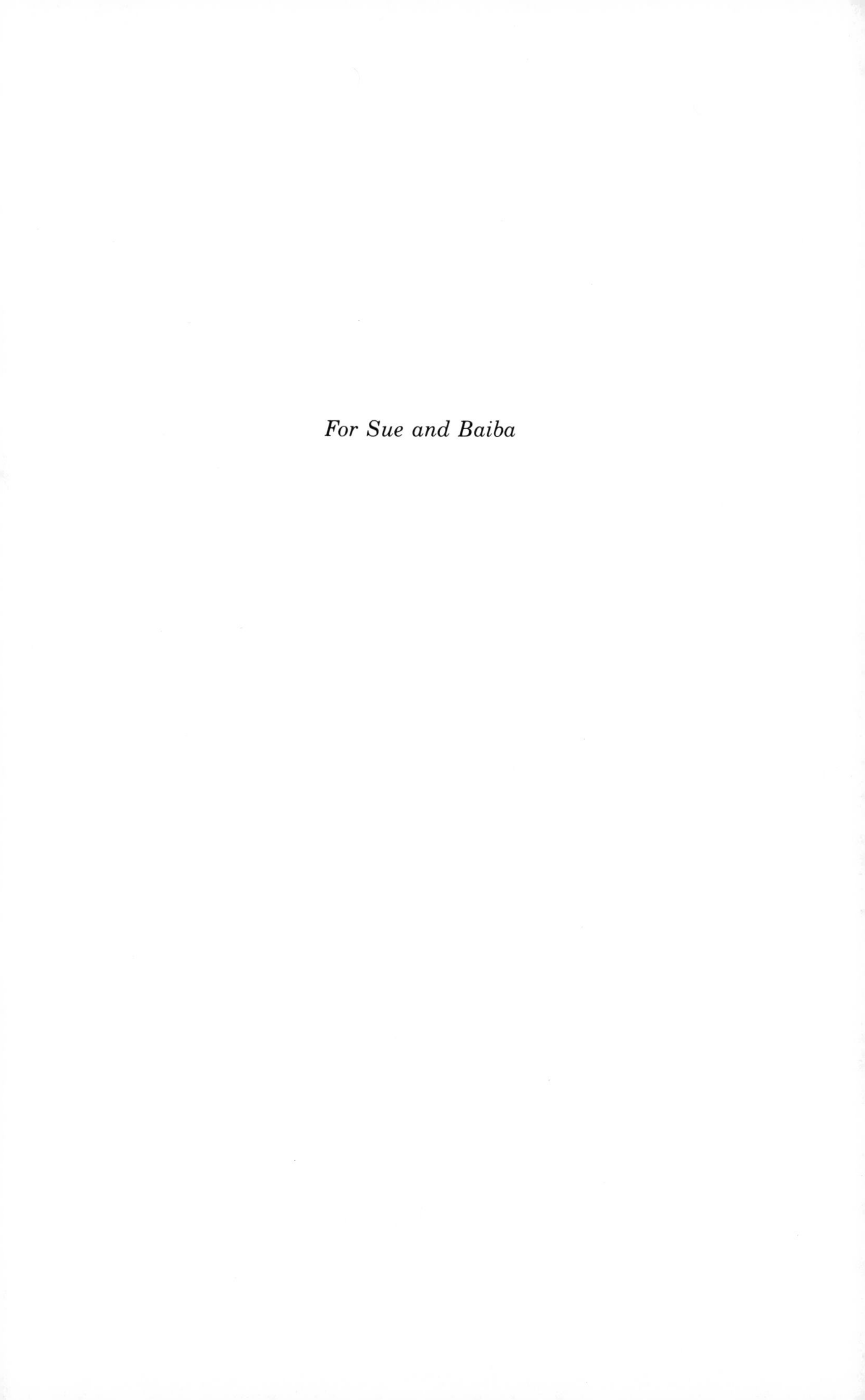

For Sue and Baiba

Contents

Introduction

Dentistry is both a technical and a person-oriented profession. The success of a practice and the satisfaction enjoyed by the dentist, the staff, and patients depend in substantial measure on how well needs and expectations can be shared and adjusted. Dentistry is more rewarding when patients understand the importance of sound personal oral hygiene or appreciate the value of the technical work performed, when staff share a common philosophy of practice, and when professionals can respond to patients' needs. These are all more likely where there is good communication. In fact, we define communication as the skill of sharing needs to create better relationships among people. Communication is a way to involve others in solving the problems we face in practicing dentistry.

Good interpersonal communication skills are essential for getting better control of what goes on in the dental office. "Getting control" involves the capacity to predict and influence the immediate environment sufficiently to get one's work done. Control implies less hassle, fewer surprises, and a greater sense of accomplishment. But unlike power, which is the unilateral manipulation of others, control benefits everybody. The dental professional who is satisfied, effective, and predictable because he or she communicates well helps both patients and coworkers get control.

The focus of this book is practical. Chapters address the most commonly occuring communication problems in the dental office, and examples are used wherever possible to illustrate the points made. The communication practices recommended are consistent with theory, even through theory has intentionally been understated. References are available in each chapter for those who wish to explore topics in detail. The communication practices recommended are also known to be effective based on the authors' experiences in dental practice and teaching.

This book is meant for students in dental, dental hygiene, and dental assisting programs. It is also designed for use in the dental office where an entire staff can use it as the foundation for a series of inservice training meetings, and selected chapters will stand alone as part of the orientation of new staff members. Teachers and practice management consultants will find the text to be a useful resource.

There are three parts in the book. The first deals with basic communication skills such as motivation, listening, and empathy. This is the fundamental repertoire common to all interpersonal relations. The second treats the way communication is used to control the relationships between patients and professionals. We call this special association based on mutual needs and expectations the "treatment alliance." There is also a "work alliance" that unifies the staff in a dental office. The communication aspects of this relationship are handled in the chapters in the third part.

Because communication is a skill, it is impossible to get much better at it without practice. The book is written to encourage active involvement. Each chapter follows a standard structure of text, a case and its analysis, references, and exercises with discussion. Because chapters focus on single basic skills or on common problems in dental practice, it is possible to use this text selectively. It is also expected that some chapters can be reviewed several times with the anticipation of improving one's skills each time. Thus, *Dental Communication* is an applied reference book.

Learning communication is different from finding out about new medications or fabricating a new appliance. Each of us already knows how to communicate, and we communicate the way we do because it suits our personality and the demands of our "work setting"—at least we have settled for the fit. To benefit from this book will require some unlearning and the questioning of an occasional personal assumption. It should definitely lead to positive changes in the practice of dentistry. It is our firm belief that, regardless of how effective one is now, communication skills can always be improved.

Part I

BASIC COMMUNICATION SKILLS

1

Characteristics of Communication

The phone rang five or six times. Beth Morris, Dr. Rose's receptionist, drummed her fingers impatiently. Finally, an answer, a groggy voice said, "Yeah . . .?"

"Uh, Mr. Forman?"

"Yeah."

"Oh, there you are. Boy, you're hard to get ahold of. I've called every day this week and I was beginning to think we'd lost you. We need to have a little chat about your balance . . ."

The voice on the other end was sharp as it interrupted, "Who is this?"

"This is Mrs. Morris at the doctor's office, where you've had your dental care. In fact, in looking over your chart here, I can see that you've had quite a bit of work done. And now you're about three months behind in your payments. Did you know that, Mr. Forman?"

There was a silence on the phone, then a resigned, "Yeah."

"Well," resumed the receptionist, "I'm sure we realize that this poses a problem. Doctor has instructed me to contact everyone with a delinquent account. Soooo . . ., Mr. Forman, the next time you come in, would you take care of your balance?"

There was no reply. "Okay?" the receptionist asked. Again a silence, then a short, "Sure, bye," and the patient hung up.

* * *

"Hi there, Mr. Forman. Before you see the Doctor, could we straighten out your account now?"

The patient hung up his coat as he answered, "Sorry about being late; got tied up with some things. Tuesday's terrible. Is Dr. Rose ready for me?"

The dentist appeared in the doorway. He smiled as he acknowledged the patient then went behind the desk. He stood close to the receptionist and in a firm voice said, "Beth, I will only be a few minutes with Mr. Forman. As soon as he leaves I want to see you in my office." Without waiting for a reply, he turned and gestured for the patient to follow him.

"Ralph, I would like to talk with you for a minute in my office." The dentist picked up the chart from the wall bracket on the way and preceded the patient into his small but very tastefully decorated office. On the walls were a large bookcase, a metal stand for storing and viewing slides, and several framed prints. The wall behind the dentist was nearly covered with framed diplomas, plaques, and letters. The desk had on it only a phone, a picture of the family, an x-ray viewbox, and about five charts.

Dr. Rose began. "I'm concerned. When you started treatment here . . ." he opened and scanned the chart ". . . five-and-a-half months ago, I thought we had an understanding about the level of care you were going to need. You have a lot of work that still needs doing, Ralph, to bring your mouth back to an ideal condition. I have really tried to do the best I could by you. As I explained, all I want is the highest quality available for all my patients, and now it seems you are drawing back a little."

The patient was ridged in the chair, gaze fixed steadily on the dentist, and motionless as he listened. Now he turned sideways abruptly, throwing one hand up in the air, as he answered sharply, "Well, what do you want, Doc? I'm here aren't I?"

The dentist continued in a calm voice. "No need to get upset. I just want to explain some things so you will understand my position." He opened the chart again and turned it toward Mr. Forman. He read the history of treatment, upside down, including payments.

Mr. Forman turned sideways again, crossed his legs and arms, stared at the chart for a moment, then absentmindedly fixed his gaze on the phone. When Dr. Rose reached Beth Morris's notation concerning the morning phone call in which back payments were discussed, the patient turned quickly and put both hands on the table. "Oh, so that's it. She's turned the collections over to you now. Well, as I explained to you a while ago, I expect to pay my bills just like everybody else, but I lost my job at the tool shop. When I told you I got the night job I thought you said it would be okay to skip a few months. Now you're putting the screws to me again."

"No, it's not that at all, Mr. Forman. You're not listening. I really am not that concerned over a few late payments. What I care about is the quality of your care. You have some serious dental problems and unless you start coming in more regularly we aren't going to be able to treat you properly. We need to work out an understanding about what needs to be done and how we're going to accomplish it." At this point, the dentist quickly reviewed the diagnosis and presented a rather extensive treatment plan.

The patient was by now passive, nodding only occasionally that he understood. Now he agreed with everything said—sometimes doing so even before Dr. Rose had completed his explanations. Eventually he moved to the edge of his seat, hands on his knees with his elbows stuck out like wings.

When the dentist was satisfied that the case had been presented in sufficient detail, he stood up. The patient followed immediately. "I'm glad we understand each other now," Dr. Rose smiled. "I think you'll be satisfied when I finish your treatment. On your way out you can make arrangements with my receptionist for the next appointment to make up for this one you missed and for a payment schedule. It was great talking to you."

* * *

Beth Morris knocked lightly on the half-open door and asked, "You wanted to see me?"

The dentist watched as the receptionist sat down, then he started in a firm, loud, steady voice; "Do you mind if I give you some feedback? You're doing a substandard job on the front desk. I hired you to handle the details of this operation so that I can do what I trained five years to do—dentistry. Your job is to keep track of appointments, insurance, charts, and payments so that we don't have problems like this fellow Forman. You've got him so upset about his payments that I wouldn't be a bit surprised if we never see him again. You've got to learn to be tactful. It took me 20 minutes to calm him down just now. And if you have any questions you can always ask, you know."

"But, Doctor," the receptionist started, "how am I supposed to know what you've told the patients. We were supposed to have a deal where you wrote everything in the treatment record, but I can't always find your comments in every case."

"Sometimes Mary (the chairside assistant) forgets," offered the dentist. "But that's no excuse. You're the one who's ultimately in charge and we can't afford this kind of problem. I just want you to do one thing for me. I want you to try harder, and I don't want you to let this kind of thing happen again. Right?"

The receptionist sat for a moment, apparently lost in thought as the dentist stared at her. Finally she looked up and said without much energy, "yeah, sure." She walked slowly out of the room.

ANALYSIS

This series of three related episodes describes communication situations that have happened in almost every office at one time or another. They also illustrate many of the points made in this book.

There are three more sections in this chapter. The first is a commentary on the three episodes, explaining in general terms what is happening as the dentist, the receptionist, and the patient communicated and how this affects each of them. This commentary references various chapters in the text. The second section is a brief analysis of the communication process in the abstract. Here are the fundamentals common to every interpersonal communication activity. The final section presents another case illustrating how Dr. Rose, Beth Morris, and Ralph Forman could talk with each other in a positive, efficient, and productive fashion.

COMMENTARY

First Episode

The initial telephone conversation is an opportunity for the receptionist to be assertive, explaining how the patient's nonpayment is creating a problem for the office and then working toward a mutually satisfactory solution. As explained in Chapter 5 (Assertiveness), this communication fails because it is too abstract and too judgmental. Chapter 4 (Power and Chauvinism) is also germane because the depersonalized language ("we" and "Doctor"), diminutives ("Have a little chat" and "Soooo . . ."), and dictating a single acceptable response without consideration of the patient express efforts to manipulate the patient's status. The predictable result in such cases is apathy (not caring) on the victim's part.

Two other chapters provide background for this episode. Compliance with Professional Suggestions (Chapter 12) explains how the dentist and the receptionist have failed to condition this patient into the habit of timely payment. Chapter 17 (Using the Telephone Effectively) contains hints on supplemental information, such as identity of the caller and the purpose of the call, that could have made the conversation more effective. That chapter also shows how to use the chart to support telephone work and avoid such awkward moments as waking a patient who works nights and sleeps in the morning.

Second Episode

The meeting in the dentist's office reflects failed communication as both Dr. Rose and Mr. Forman unsuccessfully pursue their own agendas. The dentist sought to present the treatment plan again and seemed to be asking that the patient "see things from the dentist's perspective" ("I just want to explain some things so you will understand my position," "I really tried to do the best for you," and "we need to work out an understanding").

The dentist's approach in this case fails on three grounds. First, patients' and dentists' needs are different. To maintain a relationship they must be complementary. Second, understanding does not necessarily lead to action. Finally, Dr. Rose is not being appropriately assertive. Acquiescence is the trap of ducking a situation that calls for letting others know they are causing a problem for you. Busy dentists, such as this one, frequently acquiesce ("all I want is," "I just want to explain," and "I really am not that concerned over a few late payments"). Some of the predictable consequences of acquiescence include ambiguous communication and projecting the frustration from the person causing it to the other. Other negative side effects are listed in Chapter 5.

Dr. Rose had intended this to be a persuasive meeting (Chapter 7), one designed to elicit a desired behavior and positive supporting attitudes. It had limited success because it was a monologue. Chapters 10 and 11 also pertain to this vignette. The information gathering skills detailed in the chapter on Interviewing and History Taking could have been used to diagnose this significant problem—patient reluctance to accept offered dental care. It is evident from the conversation that Treatment Planning and Informed Consent have not been well done.

The patient is trying to express his feelings. And in this short exchange he has several of them. His initial response is anger (rigid posture, punctuated by abrupt and exaggerated words and gestures) as he is upset by what he considers the dentist's violation of an informal agreement to relax the payment schedule. As the patient's anger is deflected and the dentist forces the conversation into a lecture on treatment needs, Mr. Forman grows increasingly depressed. This feeling gives way to impatience expressed by his posture and in a hollow agreement designed to expedite the presentation. Chapter 8 discusses the most common emotions encountered in the dental setting.

Dr. Rose fails to recognize these feelings, and in some cases denies them altogether ("No need to get upset" and "No, it's not that at all"). Where emotions are present to any significant extent, they must be dealt with to prevent their becoming obstacles to communication. Chapter 3 (Empathy and Rapport) explains how to identify when feelings must be addressed and how this can be done without becoming emotionally involved or "psychoanalyzing" others.

The chapter on Listening (Chapter 2) presents common barriers to hearing what others are expressing. Both patient and dentist are engaged in stereotyping and are preoccupied with what they intend to say. Neither uses any "active listening" strategies.

This episode is rich in nonverbal communication. Much of the information about Mr. Forman's feelings comes from his posture and the manner in which he speaks. The dentist, by eye contact, control of who speaks, and use of props such as the desk and chart actually creates an environment to his own liking. Additionally, the office—its furniture, the diplomas, and its supercilious order—creates a sense of control that has a strong impact on communication. These points are explored in Chapters 6 (Nonverbal Communication) and 14 (Office Environment and Written Communication).

Third Episode

The final exchange is a little staff "meeting." Like many, it is motivated by a problem and dominated by the boss. Despite his intent, Dr. Rose does not actually give feedback. Chapter 15 explains how feedback should be immediate, specific, solution-oriented, and within the responder's control. The dentist's speech is actually a general, personal judgment, with a hint of threat, and offers no assistance in either uncovering the problem or framing a solution. Chapter 16, on Intraoffice Communication, suggests that this exchange could be more effective if everyone concerned were present (chairside assistant), if all personal agenda items were on the table, and if the manager–dentist would articulate what he feels is essential in a satisfactory solution.

FUNDAMENTALS

Needs

Communication always begins with a need. When the office phone rings, we know before answering that whoever is calling is in need. When co-workers seek us out we know they want something. When patients, who normally initiate little conversation in the dental office, speak up, they are announcing an unmet need.

Most of the time people talk because they want the person with whom they are speaking to take some *action*. The dentist can obtain a clear operating field by asking the patient to turn his or her head, or with a gentle gesture. The child patient who whines, flinches, and cries may be trying to avoid a frightening part of the dental procedure. In both examples, the speakers are signaling that their needs can be met if the listener would change what he or she is doing. The speaker wants to "adjust the relationship."

But what is the need of the patient who talks incessantly with the receptionist about no topic in particular or what need lies behind the assistant's bragging about a new car? These communicators need *understanding*—an acknowledgment of their individuality or of the importance of their point of view. This is a large part of what Dr. Rose was expressing in the situation where he seeks to clarify the relationship he wants between himself and the patient.

We can thus *define communication as using words, gestures, and context to express needs with the intention of establishing or adjusting a relationship in which the listener's actions or understanding help meet the speaker's needs.*[1–6]

Hearing

It is harder to communicate than to talk because communication requires that a listener participate effectively. The speaker's needs must be heard and an appropriate response made. Thus communication is always a two-way process.[7]

The conversation in the dentist's office between Dr. Rose and Mr. Forman was frustrating because neither was listening. Expressed needs were falling on deaf ears. The symmetry in communication entails that the listener also must "need to listen." When there is no value in listening, or when expressing oneself is more important, communication stops.[8]

Hearing is a dynamic interpretation, not a literal recording of what is said.[9] Mr. Forman will only hear what suits his purpose and it will be translated into ideas that make sense in his experience. The listener's background, values, and own needs are a filter through which communication is processed. Dr. Rose is caring and articulate, but he cannot communicate until he shows concern for Mr. Forman's needs.

Communication begins with a need, but it is complete only when the speaker and listener share compatible needs and can thus establish mutually beneficial alliances.

Messages

The first of the three parts into which the book is divided presents basic communication messages—ones that express empathy and rapport, establish status, convey assertiveness, or persuade and motivate. These represent basic adjustments necessary in the alliances between dental care professionals and their patients and among co-workers.

Communication messages are like a television transmission signal that simultaneously carries code for color, pattern, and sound. The four components in a communication message, which are always present in varying degrees, include: (a) information, (b) emotion, (c) status, and (d) personality.

INFORMATION. The informational component is what could be read if the words were written and all context and nonverbal aspects stripped away. In many cases, information is dominant as in drug prescriptions, phone numbers and addresses, and consultation letters. The social patter used by dentists and staff members typically serves to keep the lines of communication open and is quickly forgotten.[10]

EMOTION. Emotions can be predominant in even the most matter-of-fact sounding statements. When Ralph Forman abruptly interjected, "Well, what do you want, Doc?" he is expressing a rather strong feeling and not asking a literal question. The dentist consistently ignored these feelings and searched for rational grounds. When emotions are a significant part of interpersonal communication they must be handled before information can be exchanged effectively,[11] hence the frustrating edge of the meeting in Dr. Rose's office.

STATUS. Communication also tells something about the status relationship that the speaker believes to exist with the listener.[12] The derogatory diminutive title, "Doc," is one obvious example. The many subtle aspects of status communication are surveyed in Chapter 4, as when the use of first names, joking around, or slang gives reliable clues to the pecking order in an office.

PERSONALITY. It is virtually impossible to separate the message from the person who expresses it.[5] The three brief episodes at the beginning of this chapter create impressions of the character of Beth Morris, Dr. Rose, and Ralph Forman. The many sample messages used in this text must be customized and will absorb the personality of the person who uses them.

Skill

Communication is a skill.[13] There are very few contexts in which it is sufficient to analyze the communication process or expound on theory. Dental care professionals must react instantly and semiconsciously to the most salient aspects of interpersonal relations and say the right things in the right way. The two parts of skill performance, identifying cues and responding to them, correspond to the two parts of communication—listening and talking.

This text has been organized to promote skill learning. Theory, though forming the foundation upon which each chapter is based, is largely buried so that actual practice is more conspicuous. Significant clues governing professional and patient interpersonal behavior are stressed at the beginning of each chapter, followed by suggested general responses. Examples and cases are thought to be more effective than explanations or rules. The exercises that conclude each chapter are strongly recommended because skills can only be learned by practice with feedback.

One special feature of learning communication skills must be mentioned to avoid possible frustration. This will be a different sort of learning from mastering intraoral instrumentation or physical evaluation of the patient. Most dental skills are new; they are an extension of the learner's capacity. Each of us, by contrast, already has developed habits of communication. These habits are firmly in place because they "work" in some sense and are self-rewarding. The techniques developed in this text will often, at first, appear to be awkward substitutes for comfortable ways. The new skills presented are grounded in theory and have been proven effective by a wide range of students. We urge that readers confirm the utility of the skills by testing their results in personal use.

REPRISE

The chapter closes with a retelling of the three episodes with which we began. The reader will notice that these new dialogues are shorter, more effective, and involve less dominance on the part of the initiator. In general it is true that experts in communication speak more frequently but use fewer words.[13] The most effective communications tend to be short, timely, and two-way.

Six months later, Beth Morris was on the phone again. "Hello, Mr. Forman? . . . This is Beth Morris in Dr. Rose's office. I just wanted to remind you about your appointment tomorrow. . . . Yes, four o'clock again." Then glancing at a note in the chart, "But I guess we're going to have to find another time after that. Dr. Rose told me you found a day job again. . . . You certainly sound happy about it. . . . See you tomorrow."

* * *

Mr. Forman was sitting in the operatory when Dr. Rose entered. "Hi, there. How do you feel this afternoon? I'll bet you're eager to see how you look with these two new crowns."

The patient nodded, "It's been a long haul getting all this work done. Looks pretty good though."

The dentist sat in front of the patient after putting some study models on the counter and turning on the viewbox. "I asked Beth to schedule you fifteen minutes early today. I wanted the chance to go over your case with you. I was looking at it after the last appointment and I think you might be as surprised as I was to compare where you were when you came in with where you are now."

Using radiographs, photographs, and models, the dentist took about five minutes to review the progress on the case. "I know you were a little uncertain at the beginning about the need for all the work we had to do."

"Well, right. It's kinda hard to admit that I let my mouth go so badly. And I'll be honest with you: I have a hard time telling what is essential and what is just nice extras, you know what I mean? There's a lot of doctors out there who don't have enough work and so they pad things. I'm not saying that you're one of them. But at the beginning, I wasn't so sure.

"You want to know what did it for me," the patient continued. "I mean what convinced me that you weren't out to rip me off? When you said you wanted my teeth to last a lifetime and you were willing to work at a pace I felt comfortable with. You know, you really scared me at the beginning. You're so organized and thorough and have everything so thought out. It's a little overwhelming. I know you didn't want to do it that way, but it really helped to take the treatment one step at a time."

"You're right, Ralph," the dentist began. "Naturally I would have preferred to finish your work more quickly. But I know you have limitations on your finances and that you wanted to see the results of the first crown before committing to more extensive treatment. But I think you can see the overall benefit now. And wait 'till you see these two crowns I have for you today . . ."

* * *

The dentist took Mr. Forman's chart to the front desk. "Here, Beth. I made some notations about Ralph Forman. I haven't heard anything about his payments. How's he coming? Can I see the ledger card?

"Ahh," said the dentist as he scanned the record of payments, "that's not too bad. How'd you accomplish that?"

"Simple," the receptionist answered as she straightened up and looked rather important. "We had a little talk about what he could afford and what we needed to run a business. At first, I think he was holding out, but once I finally got him to commit himself and then put it in writing, he's been pretty good—with a few reminders now and then."

Dr. Rose turned to return to the patient waiting for anesthesia to take effect. "Great. Keep doing it. It seems to work, and I love to catch people doing things right."

REFERENCES

1. Proceedings of the National Conference on Applied Behavioral Science. *Journal of Dental Education*, 1983, 47, entire issue.
2. Berlo, D.K. *The process of communication*. New York: Holt, Rinehart and Winston, 1960.
3. Cherry, C. *On human communication*. New York: John Wiley and Sons, 1957.
4. Patton, B.R., & Giffin, K. *Interpersonal communication in action: Basic text and readings* (2nd ed.). New York: Harper & Row, 1977.
5. Verderber, R.F. *Communicate* (2nd ed.). Belmont, Calif.: Wadsworth, 1978
6. Stewart, J., & D'Angelo, G. *Together: Communication interpersonally* (2nd ed.). Reading, Mass.: Addison-Wesley, 1980.
7. Brown, R. *Words and things*. New York: The Free Press of Glencoe, 1958.
8. Thibaut, J.W., & Kelley, H.H. *The social psychology of groups*. New York: John Wiley and Sons, 1959.
9. Bruner, J.S. *On knowing: Essays for the left hand*. Cambridge: Harvard University Press, 1962.
10. Hayakawa, S.I. *Language in thought and action*. New York: Harcourt, Brace and World, 1964.
11. Carkhuff, R.R. New training for the helping professions: Toward a technology for human and community resource development. *Counseling Psychology,* 1972, 3, 12–30.
12. Farb, P. *Word play: What happens when people talk*. New York: Bantam, 1973.
13. Cronbach, L.J. *Educational psychology* (2nd ed.). New York: Harcourt, Brace and World, 1963.

EXERCISES

1–1. Many professionals participate in study clubs and students often are members of study groups. The advantages of such "learning alliances" include faster coverage of material through division of labor, opportunity to verify one's understanding through feedback, and a supportive environment where it is safe to practice newly developed skills.

Creating such a partnership will be invaluable in mastering the communication skills presented in this book. Select a partner from your office, a fellow student, spouse, or roommate. Sit down and explain why it is important for you to learn to communicate better. Point out the benefits that your partner might expect and ask for his or her help. Together you can create a plan for the way each of you will participate in a "learning alliance." Some of the subsequent exercises in the book are written for learning partners.

1–2. Read the examples below and identify the following components of the communication process: (1) speaker's need, (2) message, and (3) desired response (action or understanding).

- **a.** Nervous looking patient to dentist: "Is this going to be a long procedure?"
- **b.** Hygienist who enters the office five minutes late to the receptionist: "What have I got first this morning?"
- **c.** Dentist to a squirming child: "I can't do a good job when you keep jumping around."

1–3. Identify an informational, emotional, and status component in each of the following messages:

- **a.** Patient to dentist: "Doctor, how much will all this stuff cost?"
- **b.** Dentist, in sympathetic voice, to assistant: "Pat, you're a little late this morning."
- **c.** Dentist to patient's mother: "The diastema and constricted palate are significant problems. I would like to refer John to an orthodontist."

DISCUSSION OF EXERCISES

1–1. This is the single most valuable exercise in the book. It is impossible to master interpersonal communication skills working alone. A sympathetic friend who is sharing your experiences is in a good position to help. Your "learning alliance" should provide opportunity for practice and feedback and supply support and encouragement. Remember that the partnership will fall apart if your helper does not perceive a personal reward for participation. Several subsequent chapters will show how this initial alliance should and can be modified as it matures.

1–2. For each example various alternatives are acceptable depending on the values and expectations of the reader and the interpretations these suggest. The following are plausible.

Speaker's Needs	*Possible Message*	*Desired Action*
a. Information to help control emotions	"I am worried about painful or dangerous procedures."	Understanding
b. Maintenance of professional relationship with patients	"Is my patient here?"	Action
c. Safe and effective working conditions	"Stop moving."	Action

1–3.

Information	*Emotion*	*Status*
a. "What will the fee be?"	"I am concerned about being able to pay for quality care."	Title shows high status for dentist
b. Reminder of obligation to be prompt	"Is everything okay?"	Voice and first name show high status and friendliness
c. "John needs orthodontic treatment."	"I care about John's oral health."	Jargon shows higher status

2

Listening

Listening forms the foundation for interpersonal communication in the dental office. It is a large part of how we learn what patients and co-workers need. Listening skills are particularly valuable in building rapport, in conducting patient and employment interviews, and for staff meetings. Because nonverbal communication also affects what we hear, we must learn to watch as part of listening.

This chapter describes the dynamics of listening and illustrates the types of errors most commonly made. A section on active listening and a section explaining how context helps and hinders perception then provide the foundation for improving listening skills.

DYNAMICS OF LISTENING

Listening is the active process of selection, generalization, and reconstruction of what we hear.[1] It is unusual to listen in a literal sense and almost impossible to avoid interpretation through our systems of needs and values. For example, consider the quotation

A bird in
the hand can be
be very messy!

and determine whether you agree with it. People whom we like and respect are generally given credit for more intelligent remarks than they actually make and their blunders are overlooked. When performing a differential diagnosis, it is dangerous to jump to conclusions because this may screen important symptoms from being heard. Now that we recognize that listening is a process of interpretation, we must look at generalizations, needs of the listener, and distractions because they influence the *interpretation* process in listening.

Generalizations versus Stereotypes

The mental categories we use to simplify our world are called generalizations.[2] When dentists hear patients complain about sensitive teeth, they listen long enough to satisfy themselves of the tentative diagnosis. All of the details about what the patient was eating, where the sensation was first noticed, and the patient's exact words fade away as useless detail leaving only the generalization that constitutes the tentative diagnosis.

Dental care would be impossible without making some simplifying generalizations. Patients with slightly different dentitions are grouped together and treated as Class II malocclusions. Some patients are said to be good candidates for preventive home care instruction or periodontal surgery despite individual variations. Similar advantages can result from knowing that a patient is a hypochondriac, mentally handicapped, or an anxious, aggressive, or depressed person. A perceptive chairside assistant and dentist will categorize children who are likely to present behavior problems and they can take preventive action as soon as the first faint cues of disruption are noticed. All of these are examples of the necessary and wise use of generalizations.

Generalizations that distort subsequent listening and that are immune to modification by reality are called stereotypes.[3] When the dentist makes a snap judgment (stereotype) that a patient is not motivated for quality care, pertinent remarks that the patient makes will not be heard or will be misinterpreted. The dentist may present a less-than-optimal treatment plan based on his or her erroneous stereotype and the patient's rejection of it will come as a surprise. An auxiliary who is stereotyped by co-workers as being "retiring and accommodating" will experience difficulty being assertive.

Needs Determine Generalizations

The generalizations we use in listening are based on our personal needs.[4] Categories such as "preventively motivated," "sensitive to pain," and "slow in making payments" are of value to dental professionals. They simplify work and direct action because they are meaningful to the dentist's and staff's needs. Most of the dental and dental auxiliary education, formal and on-the-job, is learning the meaningful categories. Good interpersonal communication skills depend on learning the useful human relations categories. For example, the patient who complained of a sensitive tooth was also expressing how he or she reacts to pain, under which conditions professional care is sought, and what is expected of professionals. The categories we have developed, based on what we value, focus what we listen to and limit what we hear. For instance, patients who do not care about plaque or find it repulsive will have a hard time identifying it. A colleague nursing a bruised ego may misperceive routine information. An anxious patient may fail to comprehend even the simplest of instructions and repeated reassurances will fall on deaf ears.

Uncontrolled Listening Leads to Distraction

The average speaking rate is 125 to 150 words per minute. Most people can absorb verbal messages at 500 to 600 words per minute. Unless we use this surplus capacity for disciplined listening, we are subject to distraction.[5] Some of these distractions include: (1) drifting or daydreaming, (2) worrying about how the conversation is going, (3) watching for a chance to interrupt, and (4) evaluating or judging what is being said. A major cause of failing to hear something important is that we have not made an opportunity for listening. We are busy with something else, we are thinking of what we want to say, or looking for a chance to break into the conversation. Sometimes we are too preoccupied in evaluating the general nature of what is being said to hear some of the important details.

The basic criterion for effective listening is making accurate and useful generalizations about what others are saying. The fundamental test is *keeping surpise to a minimum*. It is to the techniques of active listening and context checking that we now turn to learn how to reduce surprise.

ACTIVE LISTENING

Active listening means taking positive steps to insure that you interpret what the speaker is saying the way in which the speaker intends to say it.[6] It includes the three techniques of paraphrasing, verifying consequences, and preparing to listen.[7] These skills reduce the chances of a listener's surprise at the speaker's subsequent behavior, encourage the speaker, develop rapport, permit greater comprehension of details, and promptly signal when communication is breaking down.

Paraphrase Reflects Understanding

Repeating in your own words what others are saying provides an opportunity to verify that communication is accurate. Paraphrasing also shows interest and helps the listener focus and remember the most important points.

- *(Mother to dentist)* "Is it common to take out healthy teeth?" *(Active listening paraphrase—dentist to mother)* "For Jimmy's particular crowding problem, I would say so. But you seem concerned about the need to remove four permanent teeth."
- *(Assistant to dentist)* "Why do we always have to have meetings at noon?"
  (Active listening paraphrase—dentist to assistant) "I guess you don't think it's fair to have staff meetings on your lunch time?"

It may be noted in these examples that more than the literal message is being reflected. In both cases the dentist amplifies the message in a tentative fashion hoping to capture in words the emotional component as well as the literal one.

Verifying Consequences Confirms Requests

Another method of active listening uses the consequences of a request or statement. If the dentist requests a full-mouth series of radiographs on a patient, the assistant could question (silently), ""Is this a new patient?" Adding detailed examples is another means of confirming that the speaker's point has been correctly grasped.

- *(Receptionist to dentist)* "Doctor, we're having a lot of trouble with preauthorization lately"
  (Active listening for consequences—dentist to receptionist) "Right, we're still holding on to Mr. Barber, and that big bridge case probably is not back yet either, is it?"

Preparation Improves Listening

Often listening can be made more effective with a little preparation. This means thinking through what a person is likely to say before you meet him or her, thus freeing yourself of distractions such as charts and competing thoughts. Sometimes this means placing yourself in a position to observe the nonverbal components of communication or just to hear better. Sometimes it is necessary to get the speaker's cooperation.

- *(Hygienist to patient)* "That sounds unusual, Mrs. Odell. Let me finish taking your blood pressure and then I want to hear all about that rash."
- *(Receptionist to dentist)* "Okay, can I finish getting this insurance information and then take the supply orders?" (A question has been asked, wait for a reply.)
- *(One assistant to another)* "I only have a minute before the next patient. This sounds like something really important. Do you want to talk about it at lunch?"

CONTEXT CHECKING

Every speech has a message and a context.[8] Usually the message is information and the context is how and where the communication takes place. In fact, what is message and what is context depend on the interests of the listener and may change depending on circumstances. For example, count the number of times the word "be" appears in the quotation on page 17. Many people miss the extra word when reading for content as you were asked to do when the quote was introduced.

When messages sound phony, surprising, meaningless, humorous, or awkward it is because they do not fit their context. In these instances there is some inconsistency between the information coming from the patient or co-worker and (1) the nonverbal communication, (2) the situation, (3) the status of the speaker, or (4) the emotional tone of the message. When the patient winces while reporting that everything is fine, this is a signal to investigate further. When the receptionist asks the dentist who is hanging around the front desk if everything is alright and the dentist mumbles, "Oh, yeah, sure," it is possible that something is being left unsaid. Patients who relate only the factual part of a story about a traumatic situation are often holding back.

A good listener cannot attend to both the message and the context with equal concentration. Attention is generally focused on the dental information from patients or the work-related comments of co-workers, while the back of one's mind is semiconsciously aware of the fit between message and context. Whenever a message seems out of context, it should be treated as suspect and later verified.

Nonverbal Context

Inflection, pauses, eye contact, posture, and facial expressions all amplify or modify what is being said. Note the inconsistency in the following example. The chairside assistant asks the dentist whether it is alright to leave a few minutes early and the dentist grumbles without eye contact, "Na, . . . go ahead." In this case, the stated fact that the dentist does not mind is out of character with the feelings expressed by the nonverbal components of communication.

Situational Context

How should a new patient behave or what is appropriate behavior for a job applicant, a staff member called into the dentist's private office, or a patient who has just been given bad news? If the speech of these people is bouncy and light, it is likely that they are covering some insecurities and a literal interpretation of what they say thus would be hazardous.

Relational Context

Every message has a status component, and there is an implied relationship between the speaker and the listener. Are patients talking about family health history in excruciating detail because they think you need this information for professional purposes or because they find you to be a sympathetic listener? Is your fellow worker explaining intimacies of his or her personal life out of a feeling that a relationship between colleagues requires this or in the belief that your relationship is more personal? Without correctly perceiving the relationship the speaker believes to exist, the listener is likely to miss part of the message.

Emotional Context

Because messages contain both an emotional and an informational component, it is useful to know which the speaker is trying to emphasize. This involves knowledge of the speaker, the nonverbal messages, and the relationship, and selectively switching focus back and forth between feelings and thoughts, searching for the interpretation that contains the most meaning.

Consider the following examples that are rather ambiguous when taken out of context.

- *(Assistant to hygienist)* "It's five o'clock. Time to go."
  Emotional nonverbals: Assistant stands facing hygienist with hands on hips.
  Informational nonverbals: Assistant sticks head around corner, does not wait for reply.
- *(Patient to dentist)* "How much will all this cost?"
  Emotional situation: New patient has listened impassively to an involved case presentation.
  Informational situation: Patient of several years has just heard two treatment plans compared.
- *(Receptionist to patient)* "We have a policy in this office of charging a nominal fee for broken appointments when we are not notified in advance."
  Emotional relationship: Patient is a friend and has a history of "no shows."
  Informational relationship: New patient has inquired about financial matters.

CASE: THE PATIENT WITH TWO IDENTITIES

"Tell me something about Jenny's dietary habits, Mrs. Arnold," the hygienist said as she turned to face the well-dressed and articulate mother. But then without pausing, the hygienist, Anne Whitely, continued, "What does she usually have for breakfast?"

The hygienist continued her series of questions for about five minutes, commenting on each response. "Oh, I see," "That's good . . . great," "Oh, oh. That's a lot of fermentable carbohydrates, don't you think?" Finally she concluded, "Well, that about does it. I expect you do try to control between-meal snacks since you obviously care about Jenny's health." Mrs. Arnold barely had time to nod agreement when Anne Whitely continued, "There's nothing really out of the ordinary for a family like yours. Do you have any questions before we go on to some recommendations for improving Jenny's diet?"

Mrs. Arnold was looking at her daughter and answered in a distant voice, "Well, no." Then she added rather quickly, "I'm a little confused by all this. I brought Jennifer in for a routine cleaning and examination. All we have had so far are x-rays and some questions. You seem very knowledgable, Miss Whitely, but Jennifer has never seen you before and I didn't know that I wasn't giving her the right kind of diet."

"Oh, don't worry. I can tell that you are the kind of parent who wants the best for Jenny. And that's why I'm taking the time to go over this important information with you. Now let me just make a few recommendations . . ."

Anne's brief summary of the relationship between food, plaque, and caries was clear and logical. She suggested some minor and easy modifications in diet and then asked again for questions. This time Mrs. Arnold was more direct. "Fine. Now are you going to clean Jennifer's teeth?"

ANALYSIS

In this example, two intelligent women who both care about the child's dental health fail to communicate because neither can listen to the needs the other is expressing. The mother, who calls her daughter Jennifer, needs to feel like a good parent. The hygienist, who calls the patient Jenny, needs to feel like an effective dental educator. By the end of the dialogue both women feel frustrated, misunderstood, and perhaps angry. If Anne Whitely expects that Mrs. Arnold will follow her good advice, she will be surprised and disappointed.

It is appropriate to discuss diet, but the hygienist should first confirm that the parent is informed about the procedures planned for the appointment. "Mrs. Arnold, do you and Jennifer know what we plan to do and discuss today?" This would provide an opening for the mother to state her concerns.

Unfortunately, the hygienist focused on the informational content in Mrs. Arnold's messages without apparent sensitivity to the context. She was unaware of the importance of the situation (Mrs. Arnold had brought her child for a prophylaxis). The two women appear to have defined their relationship differently (Mrs. Arnold used formal names and protested that she had never seen the new hygienist before). The nonverbal cues, such as no eye contact and very slow reponses when denying that there were other questions, show that Mrs. Arnold's verbal messages were not to be taken literally. When Mrs. Arnold explained her expectations for the visit and questioned Anne Whitely's credibility, she signaled that she wanted her emotional needs attended to. The hygienist brushed them aside with, "Oh, don't worry."

Anne Whitely stereotyped the mother. "You obviously care about Jenny's health" and "There's nothing out of the ordinary for a family like yours" are verbal expressions that the hygienist sees this family as excellent candidates for dietary counseling. That stereotype was never verified and it controlled both what Anne Whitely said and what she heard. It would be safe to assume that Mrs. Arnold has stereotyped the hygienist, and it would be surprising if the stereotype was flattering.

REFERENCES

1. Bruner, J.S. On perceptual readiness. *Psychological Review*, 1957, 64, 123–152.
2. Vernon, M.D. *The psychology of perception*. Baltimore: Penguin, 1962.
3. Brown, R. *Social psychology*. New York: The Free Press, 1965.
4. Bruner, J.S. Social psychology and perception. In E. Maccoby, T.M. Newcomb, & E.L. Hartley (Eds.); *Readings in social psychology*. New York: Holt, Rinehart & Winston, 1958.
5. Egan, G. *Encounter: Group process for interpersonal growth*. Monterey, Calif.: Wadsworth, 1970.
6. Verderber, R.F. *Communicate* (2nd ed.). Belmont, Calif.: Wadsworth, 1978.
7. Nichols, R.G. Do we know how to listen? Practical help in a modern age. *Speech Teacher*, 1961, 10, 120.
8. Kohler, W. *Gestalt psychology: An introduction to new concepts in modern psychology*. New York: The New American Library, 1947.

EXERCISES

2–1. Perform a surprise inventory of your value structure. Carry a few 3 x 5 cards in your pocket or handbag for a week. Each time you find something unexpected, awkward, or surprising, note it on the cards. At the end of the week, review the cards to see if there are areas that continuously reoccur.

2–2. Taking notes when listening to a lecture or doing a patient interview is a form of active listening. Making marginal notes or underlining while reading is "active reading." If you are currently reading actively, switch to the passive mode for the next chapter. If you are now reading without a pencil, get one and underline as you read the next chapter. Compare what you retain reading actively and passively.

2–3. Proper sensitivity to context can enhance accurate listening. Try intentionally distorting the context and observe how rapidly communication deteriorates. Practice explaining something important or interesting to you in an emotionless voice and without facial expression. Deliver the message to a friend.

2–4. Put a piece of clean adhesive tape on a window. Position yourself so that the tape is seen against a dark background such as a building or a tree. Move so that the tape is now seen against a light background such as the sky. The tape will seem to change color.

2–5. Review the surprise inventory you made in Exercise 2-1. Can you recall the circumstances well enough to remember whether the messages were inconsistent with their context.

DISCUSSION OF EXERCISES

2–1. The surprise inventory usually reveals that there are certain areas or people associated with recurrent surprises, perhaps a co-worker or spouse, maybe current events or human nature in general. These are areas where attention could improve relationships. Often there is a strained relationship that hinders communication. It is unusual for the list of surprises to contain information about our own behavior—our dental work if we are dentists, hygienists, or students or our telephone behavior if we use the telephone frequently. These are such important activities that we have either developed useful generalizations or there is a great deal of survival value in the stereotypes that prevent our accurately perceiving the unexpected.

2–2. Most people remember better and can use more of the material they read when they actively try to identify the key points or make comments in the margin. If you would like to receive the benefits of an even more active reading skill, review your underlining quickly at the end of each section and mentally or in writing list the key points.

2–3. The usual response is some confusion on the part of the listener. This will be shown by the listener's nonverbals or perhaps even a question such as, "what's wrong?" Often the conversation will simply be allowed to drop because the listener does not know how to proceed.

2–4. By moving so that the tape is near the border between the light and dark backgrounds and alternately closing one then the other eye, the effect can be very pronounced. The perceived color change, which is real, is a result of the interaction between object and context.

2–5. If several examples do not spring to mind, perhaps you may want to repeat the surprise inventory above, paying particular attention to context.

3

Empathy and Rapport

This chapter is about listening and responding to others' feelings. Building rapport and trust, sensing how patients and co-workers feel, and letting them know that you care can improve virtually all aspects of dental practice. The goal is not to spend a lot of time discussing emotions, but one needs to know when and how to do this. The chapter first presents rapport, the harmonious relationships among people that make communication easier, and then empathy is discussed. Empathy is a special way of listening and responding to people who are trying to tell you how they feel. On a percentage basis, very little of dental communication involves developing rapport or responding empathically. But when this vital foundation is neglected, all communication is compromised.

RAPPORT—THE HELPING RELATIONSHIP

In the health professions it is not enough to know how to help people; the *right* to do so must also be earned.[1] An old saying summarizes this well: "No one cares how much you know until they know how much you care." It is documented that a foundation of patient–professional rapport is valuable for effective therapy. Dental phobia, myofacial pain, and postsurgical pain relief all respond to a trusting and open relationship between patient and dentist.[2–4] Because patients are generally incapable of judging the technical quality of the work dentists perform, the rapport that comes from relating on a person-to-person basis is a significant part of their definition of quality of care.

Characteristics of Rapport

Rapport is a mutual sense of openness, trust, and spontaneity, an absence of defensiveness and freedom from censored speech.[5] Without defensiveness, communication can be complete across the full range of information, emotions, status, and personality. This fullness of communication makes dentistry easier. Another advantage of rapport is the trust it entails. Mutual credit is extended; each action need not be justified.[6] This results in smoother, more efficient treatment and will save several times over the initial investment in establishing rapport.

Rapport is reciprocal. Although one person may take the initiative, both parties must agree on the level of openness to be maintained. Professionals have to be willing to listen to a mother's theory on teenage snack behavior or a 70-year-old's views on denture fit if they expect to have their own advice heeded. Rapport should not be confused with liking another person. Liking is not necessarily reciprocal and often fosters selective communication calculated to be ingratiating.

A pleasant and effective dental office will foster both professionalism and rapport. These concepts are complementary, not inconsistent. Professional respect is based on an appreciation of the dentist's and the staff's technical abilities; rapport is based on respect for people. When professionalism is absent, patients express their mixture of fear and contempt in excessive familiarity, which damages rapport. Conversely, poor rapport generates a defensiveness that undermines professionalism.

Establishing Rapport

Rapport is a positive response to the whole person, not just to what they are saying. One way of showing this is to give back to others more than mere social convention dictates. This is a common theme in the five techniques for establishing rapport shown in Table 3–1.

Part of being personal includes a willingness to engage in small talk. Interpersonal relations are emphasized because the information in what is being said lacks significance. Chatting about vacations, new clothes, the fortunes of the local high school football team, or the patient's children communicates a general interest in what others have to say. Such uncontroversial and

TABLE 3–1. FIVE TECHNIQUES FOR ESTABLISHING RAPPORT

A teenager is expressing apprehension over having to wear braces. "How do you think I will look?"

Technique	Function	Example
Personal	Shows interest in the whole person	"You will look as pretty with braces as you do now without them."
Nontechnical	Willingness not to stress status differences	"Judging appearances is a personal thing. What do you think?"
Humorous	Spontaneity and impression of uncensored expression	"Oh, gee. I just put braces on several guys who would love to meet you."
Volunteered information	Willingness to communicate beyond mere requirements of courtesy	"Let me tell you about several girls like you who have braces now."
Identify with other	Sharing common interests	"My daughter is about your age and she has braces too."

nonthreatening topics are particularly valuable as ways of starting a conversation.

Avoiding technical language is a sound way to build rapport when status differences exist. When only dental topics are discussed, the professional's status is emphasized. When a willingness is indicated to talk about cars, hair styles, skiing, and television personalities, dental professionals add a new and personal dimension to the relationship.

Professionals who are willing to laugh at themselves or to chance a little humor demonstrate a secure sense of self-worth. Spontaneous humor is most effective because it shows that communication is not being censored.

Volunteer information and encourage others to do so. No rapport can be developed when communication is limited to the minimal responses required to be civil. Patients who answer all questions with "yes" or "no" need to be drawn out. An excellent gauge of the depth of rapport developed is the extent to which patients are willing to volunteer information not required.

Rapport can also be built through searching for and emphasizing common likes and dislikes.[7] If a patient is enthusiastic about new lower air fares, the dental professional can find something good in this news. If someone is depressed by the rain, reflecting on how it is also getting you down helps build rapport. How can patients disagree with the professional advice of a dentist who has shown such good taste by criticizing the universally hated sewer tax and complimenting the academic scholarship of the patient's daughter?

Gestures, posture, and other nonverbal communication are helpful in establishing rapport.[8] Individuals who have an open and trusting relationship are more demonstrative in their expression, make more eye contact, and are closer together when they talk.

The dentist's personal preferences, circumstances, and local and regional norms all require adjustments in the amount of casual conversation that is appropriate. Overdoing the length or familiarity of informal discussions can raise questions about professionalism, particularly when the patient is impatient. It is not the quantity of chitchat that matters. What counts is indicating a willingness to relate on a personal basis as a supplement to normal professional relations; this can be accomplished in a few sentences.

- *(Dentist to patient)* "Hi. What's new since I saw you last March?" (Permits the patient to choose a dental complaint or a personal matter.)
- *(Hygienist to child patient)* "That's a pretty dress. Is it new?" (Pride and maturity need to be reinforced in all patients, but particularly in children. This message communicates respect.)
- *(Dentist to front desk staff)* "If this last patient is a 'no-show' by quarter 'till, I'm going shopping. This has certainly been a terrible day, hasn't it?" (It is acceptable for staff members to share feelings of fatigue and frustration but it is unprofessional to communicate these to patients except under special circumstances.)

EMPATHY

There are two aspects to the skill of communicating empathy. The first is attempting to understand others from their own perspective without losing one's own identity and objectivity. The second aspect is reflecting back this understanding in ways that help others solve their own problems.[9] Consider the problem of dealing with a distant, calculating, and silent patient during a case presentation. The issues are: (1) how to bring the patient's disruptive feelings into the open so that the patient can handle them without becoming defensive, (2) how the professional can show warmth and caring without taking over responsibility for the patient's feelings, and (3) which words will lead to better dental care and rapport between dentist and patient. The next three sections address these problems in succession.

How to Respond With Empathic Understanding

Responses of empathic understanding have the following characteristics:[10]

1. They accurately reflect others' feelings.
2. They connect the feelings to concrete circumstances that are likely to be causing the feelings.
3. They accept the feelings as real and important.
4. They are nonjudgmental—they do not compromise the listener's objectivity.

The examples of empathy that follow all have these characteristics. In addition, it should be noticed that the responses are short and they encourage a further response from the person whose emotions are causing the problem. Timing, tone of voice, facial expressions, and other nonverbel components of communication are very important when expressing empathy.

- *(Hygienist to patient who winces when told that a full-mouth series of radiographs need to be taken)* "You seem concerned about the need for these x-rays."
- *(Dentist to child who refuses to open his mouth)* "Perhaps you are afraid I will try to trick you and do something you don't like."
- *(Assistant to dentist who is scowling at the day sheet and looking at his watch)* "Something about the day sheet seems to be bothering you."

For people who are just learning how to communicate empathically, it is often awkward to use nonjudgmental paraphrases. "What good," they ask, "can it do for a dentist to say 'you seem concerned' to a patient who is very obviously concerned?" The answer is that it typically does a world of good. The literal message is not what matters. Communicating understanding by means of a nonjudgmental paraphrase also expresses three other important messages:

- "I care how you feel."
- "I am trying to understand how you feel."
- "It is alright with me if you feel as you do."

When to Respond with Empathy

Timing is critical to the effectiveness of empathy. The rule is: When the emotional component appears to be a significant part of what others are saying it is time to try reflecting these feelings. Emotions, when they are present to any appreciable extent, predominate over and alter attempts at normal exchange of information.

Sometimes only the tip of an emotional iceberg may be revealed. Patients and co-workers express a small concern as a trial balloon or bury their emotions in seemingly informational messages in order to learn whether their feelings will be recognized and respected. When unsure, an empathic response is quite easy and safe. It is better to be safe than sorry and others are usually flattered that you care about their feelings even when it turns out that there are no problems.

- *(Patient to dentist)* "How long will this procedure take?"
  (Plausible translation) "Is this a serious or painful procedure?"
  (Poor response) "Oh, not too long. Just relax."
  (Appropriate response) "This procedure seems to be bothering you."
- *(Dentist to assistant)* "You're leaving early, humm?"
  (Plausible translation) "Why are you leaving so early when you haven't checked with me?"
  (Poor response) "Gee, I guess I forgot to tell you. I have to get to the court house before five to file a form."
  (Appropriate response) "Oh, oh. I'll bet you're upset because I didn't tell you that I have to leave early."

As difficult as it may appear, empathy is also an effective response when strong emotions are directed personally at us. Exaggerated displays of emotion are often triggered when people sense that their feelings are being ignored. The message in a scowl, a tantrum, or a threat is "You must acknowledge and accept the way I feel as a minimal condition for returning to normal communication." It is silly to ignore emotions that are so strong or to deny their importance by being rational. It is also inappropriate to acknowledge the feelings and leave it at that.

Acknowledge strong emotions with an empathic message and then set realistic limits on behavior.[11]

- *(Assistant to hygienist)* "Boy, you are upset. I had no idea you were so concerned about those curettes (states other's feeling and probable cause). I guess I don't know what you want. We had better go over the whole procedure (sets rational limits)."
- *(Dentist to young patient)* "I realize this is an uncomfortable procedure and it has been a long time (states other's feelings and probable cause). But you must keep your head still and you must not raise your arms because that could cause injury (sets rational limits)."
- *(Receptionist on phone to patient who is shouting for instant relief)* "Oh, Mr. Lawton, I know that the pain must be awful. The day after surgery is sometimes worse. It must hurt terribly (much empathy). Can you wait a minute while I try to get Dr. Biddle? (question asked so wait for an answer). He is with a patient, I will be right back to talk with you myself (set realistic expectations)."

Useless and Damaging Responses

In situations where emotions should be handled, some responses are as useless as trying to ignore the situation and some are worse.[6,11] The aim of empathic understanding is to bring out feelings that are preventing optimal treatment and to do this in a context where the patient or co-worker can assume responsibility for their own feelings. Simply saying that you "understand" requires faith on the other's part. Giving advice ignores feelings and draws attention away from the person with the problem. Pointed questioning and presuming to know how others feel invite defensive cutting of communication lines. Examples of these poor strategies are shown in Table 3–2.

Avoid phrases such as "don't worry" and "everything is going to be alright." As strange as it may sound, reassurance is damaging in most situations involving emotions. It denies others' feelings, shifts responsibility to the professional, may imply a promise that cannot be kept, and limits communication.[10]

Imagine for a minute that you are a frightened or angry patient or employee. What do the following messages communicate about the importance of your feelings?

- *(Dentist to assistant who is asking about changing hours)* "No sweat; we'll work something out for sure." (Possible

TABLE 3–2. UNWISE RESPONSES TO EMOTIONAL SITUATIONS

Poor Response	Example of Poor Response	Example of Better Response
Presumption	"I see you're obviously confused about the treatment plan." (Judgmental, implies patient is slow to comprehend)	"You seem uncertain about the treatment plan." (Describes appearances, invites patient response)
Interrogating	"Why are you so nervous?" (Implied superiority, may lead to dead-end denial)	"Not knowing what to expect can make you nervous." (Patient can agree without self-incrimination)
Abstract	"I understand how you must feel." (Patient must take your word, shifts attention away from patient)	"You seem surprised by the fee." (Shows that you understand and allows chance for correction)
Advice	"Here's what I would do . . ." (Responds on intellectual level, draws attention to you)	"It sounds like you have a very tough decision." (Indicates interest and willingness to help without taking over problem)
Reassurance	"Oh, don't worry. Everything always turns out fine." (Denies importance of other's feelings, makes promise that may not be possible to keep)	"The thought of this surgery seems to bother you." (Opens discussion of a topic very much on patient's mind)

interpretation: "The problem is too trivial for me to worry about now.")

- *(Hygienist to patient who remarks about blood on the napkin)* "That's nothing to worry about; it's normal." (Possible interpretation: "I'm busy cleaning teeth. Don't bother me with your concerns.")
- *(Dentist to patient who asks what will be involved in the surgery)* "It's routine." (Possible interpretation: "I hope this turns out 'okay' and I don't want the patient to know any more than is necessary.")

CASE: DORTMUNDER'S SUSPENDED SENTENCE

A man came briskly into the busy office. He walked immediately to the reception window, put both hands on the counter and interrupted the receptionist who was on the telephone to say, "Hi, I'm Frank Dortmunder. I don't have an appointment but I need to see Dr. Short. I've got a terrible toothache. Can you . . ."

Without looking up or covering the telephone, the receptionist, Alice Baker, interrupted, "I'm sorry. As you can see, we're very busy.

So if you will wait just a minute I'll take care of you."

Rather than taking a seat, Mr. Dortmunder turned around and leaned on the counter. He sighed repeatedly, shifted his weight from foot to foot in exaggerated impatience. Finally, Alice Baker was so embarrassed that she cut short the telephone call and said, "Now, sir, what can we do for you?"

Mr. Dortmunder began to repeat his request and the receptionist interrupted again, "I'm sorry, but the Doctor does not see emergencies in the afternoon. I can give you an appointment for tomorrow morning or I have a list of other dentists in town who might be able to work you in on such short notice."

Mr. Dortmunder looked flustered. "What? What kind of a dental office is this when you won't even help a man with a toothache? I've been coming to this guy, Short, for three years and you'd think . . ."

"Oh, I'm sorry, sir," Alice put in. "You didn't say you were a patient-of-record. I will find your chart. Just one minute," and she left.

The frustrated patient paced in a very small circle in front of the reception window. As he did so, the part-time receptionist, Karen McDonald, came into the reception area. "Hi, is someone helping you?" she asked.

"Not so's you'd notice," Mr. Dortmunder answered. "Some lady's looking for my records so she can bill me or something and she tells me I can't even see the dentist. I've got a toothache."

"Yes, I can see why you are frustrated if you think that no one will take care of you."

"Well, like I told that other one, I've got a toothache and I've been coming here for three years."

"I see your tooth really hurts. I'm sure we'll be able to give you some kind of help. I'm Karen McDonald. What is your name?"

"Dortmunder, Frank Dortmunder. I've been coming here for years."

"I'm sure," the assistant said as she reached for the day sheet, "that Dr. Short will not let you leave the office without examining you. How long has this tooth been bothering you, Mr. Dortmunder?"

ANALYSIS

Here is a brief example of the power of messages that communicate empathic understanding. Compared to the response he gave to Alice Baker, Mr. Dortmunder was much more civil with the empathic Karen McDonald. The major difference is that Alice responded only to the information component in the patient's communication. Karen responded to both the emotional and the informational part of his message, and she responded to the feelings first.

A number of clues suggest that Mr. Dortmunder's feelings

were of significance. First, it is safe to assume that anyone entering a dental office has a higher than normal emotional level. Next, it is wise to remember that people making requests are vulnerable and this patient's request is unusual. Finally, Mr. Dortmunder signaled the importance of his feelings by his brusque and forward behavior.

Besides ignoring Mr. Dortmunder's feelings, Alice Baker committed several other tactical communication errors. Her judgmental remarks ("as you can see we're busy" and "such short notice") provoke a defensive reaction from the patient. Every response from the receptionist began with the phrase "I'm sorry," but her formal manner, her interruption of the patient three times, and her use of dental jargon ("patient-of-record") communicated the opposite of warmth and respect.

Alice Baker also failed to use anyone's name: her own, the patient's (sir), or Dr. Short's (Doctor). The impression she creates of Dr. Short is that of a nameless and distant individual who lays down policy but has no time for people. Contrast this with the view one receives of Dr. Short from Karen McDonald. Dr. Short is a real and caring individual who wants to relieve the patient's pain.

Karen McDonald responds to Mr. Dortmunder's feelings with messages that show empathy and build rapport. She reflects his most obvious emotions first ("Yes, I can see why you are frustrated"). She ties these feelings to a concrete situation ("you think that no one will take care of you"). She is nonjudgmental and acknowledges that it is appropriate to feel frustrated. She also avoids questioning Mr. Dortmunder about his feelings. Her second comment is similarly empathic ("I see your tooth really hurts"). This simple statement also communicates warmth and shows that Karen McDonald cares how Mr. Dortmunder feels.

Obviously Mr. Dortmunder is more demanding and abrasive than a patient should be. His behavior toward Alice Baker is in poor taste. But Alice's defensive response is also unfortunate. It invites a spiral of bad feeling. More importantly, it is unprofessional. The role of all health care professionals is to render care. It is not to pass judgment on patients, no matter how obnoxious they may be.

REFERENCES

1. Brammer, L.M. *The helping relationship: Process and skills.* Englewood Cliffs, New Jersey: Prentice-Hall, 1973.
2. Egbert, L., Battit, G., Welch, C., & Bartlett, M. Reduction in postoper-

ative pain by encouragement and instruction of patients. *New England Journal of Medicine*, 1964, 270, 825–827.

3. Kleinknecht, R.A., Klepac, R.K., & Alexander, L.D. Origins and characteristics of fear of dentistry. *Journal of the American Dental Association*, 1973, 86, 842–848.
4. Laskin, D.M., & Greene, C.S. Influence of the doctor–patient relationship on placebo therapy for patients with myofacial–pain–dysfunction (MPD) syndrome. *Journal of the American Dental Association*, 1972, 85, 892-894.
5. Miller, GR., & Steinberg, M. *Between people: A new analysis of interpersonal communication*. Chicago: Science Research Associates, 1975.
6. Gazda, G.W., Walters, R.P., & Childers, W.C. *Human relations development: A manual for health sciences*. Boston: Allyn and Bacon, 1975.
7. Brown, R. *Social psychology*. New York: The Free Press, 1965.
8. Knapp, M.L. *Nonverbal communication in human interaction* (2nd ed.). New York: Holt, Rinehart and Winston, 1978.
9. Rogers, C.R. *On becoming a person*. Boston: Houghton Mifflin, 1961.
10. Carkhuff, R.R. New training for the helping professions: Toward a technology for human and community resource development. *Counselling Psychology*, 1972, 3, 12–30.
11. Gordon, T. *P.E.T. in action*. New York: Bantam Books, 1976.

EXERCISES

3–1. A patient is sitting in the chair immediately following the extraction of a single impacted third molar. He says, "Thanks, Doc, that really wasn't so bad. But my roommate says that the rough part is tonight. What if these pills you gave me aren't strong enough?" Comment on each of the following responses:

a. "I understand and sympathize with you."

b. "You're not worried by a story like that, are you?"

c. "You don't need to be concerned. I chose exactly the proper dosage."

Now write a response that shows empathic understanding.

3–2. Can you identify significant emotional components in the following messages?

a. (Patient to hygienist) "Is all this plaque control stuff really that effective?"

b. (Part-time to full-time receptionist) "How do you cope with all this insurance paperwork?"

c. (Dentist to staff) "There's never anyone around when you need them."

3–3. Pick one time, such as Thursday at four o'clock, to practice empathic understanding for just one hour. At the end of the hour stop and reflect back on your experiences.

3–4. Identify a close friend or co-worker (or your learning partner) with whom you share the openness, trust, and spontaneity of rapport. Think back to the last several times you met. List on a piece of paper as many characteristics of your communication as possible.

DISCUSSION OF EXERCISES

3–1. The first response requires that the patient place faith in the dentist without giving any reason to do so. Tone of voice will have a great deal to do with its effectiveness, but the words themselves are of limited value. The second approach will do more harm than good. It denies the importance of the patient's feelings and questions the patient's intelligence. The final alternative also denies the legitimacy of the patient's concerns and terminates conversation. A useful response that shows empathy and invites constructive discussion would be something like the following: "You seem worried about the possibility of not being able to get sufficient pain relief after you have left the office."

3–2. It is possible to find many suggested emotions in such apparently innocent questions or statements. The context and the nonverbal component of the messages are very important. Some plausible interpretations include: (a) "Am I getting taken?" (b) "Help me; I don't think I can cope." (c) "I'm upset at having to carry more than my share of the work."

3–3. Choosing a specific, limited time to work on skills is more likely to be successful than making a general resolve to do so. It also helps to have a friend who is working on a similar project with whom you can compare notes.

3–4. Your list should include many of the types of messages in Table 3–1. Some people use only a few of the techniques for developing rapport. Our styles reflect our personalities and our emotional needs.

4

Power and Chauvinism

Almost every message reflects something of the status relationship that exists between the speaker and the listener. Many patients show respect by using titles such as Doctor and avoiding personal or humorous topics when talking to the dentist. Sometimes a conscious effort is made to gain favor by inflating the listener's status through flattery. Generally, the status dimension of communication forms part of the semiconscious background and we become aware of it only when it is grossly out of character with the expected relationship.

Although semiconscious, status profoundly influences both interpersonal relations, as expressed in terms of power, and the communication process. When intentional or unintentional "put downs" cause alienation and disrupted communication, we are speaking of linguistic chauvinism.

The way we express and respond to status in communication is very deeply ingrained in our personality. Both chauvinism and feminism are learned communication habits, and they are resistant to change because they reflect the individual's basic needs and values.[1] What has been learned can be unlearned, and the first two steps are to become sensitive to the role of status in communication and to observe its effects.

This chapter is divided into four sections. Power, the legitimate basis for differences in interpersonal relations, is discussed first. Then artificial manipulations of status through language, what we call chauvinism, is detailed. The consequences of chauvinism and its opposite, respect for others, are explained in the third section. Finally, some positive status changing communications are presented.

POWER

Power is the capacity to get others to do things they might not otherwise do.[2] It is a legitimate basis for differences in influence and status among people. A patient who is suing for malpractice can, for example, make the dentist review and copy records, retain a lawyer, and appear for hearings. The receptionist can give one hygienist all the problem patients and thus make him or her work harder. The dental supply salesman with a unique product can demand high prices and appointment times that are inconvenient for the dentist. Some of the speech patterns characteristic of persons with high status and power are listed in Table 4–1.

Power is derived from three sources: position, expertise, and having something others want. It is enhanced by communication skills.

Position

Sometimes interpersonal influence resides in a position, title, or job, regardless of who occupies it. Society has assigned a high status to American dentists and their position is sanctioned and codified in state dental practice acts that reserve special powers to dentists. If an assistant has assigned status because the dentist has made that employee responsible for a task such as ordering

TABLE 4–1. SPEECH ATTRIBUTES OF PERSONS WITH HIGH STATUS

Speak first
Are seldom interrupted
Initiate more jokes and personal topics of conversation
Make more requests and ask more questions
Speak more slowly and in a louder voice
Pause longer between topics
Maintain greater eye contact while talking and less when listening
Are addressed more often by title or first and last name
Make more and larger gestures
Use slang or coarse speech but are less likely to hear it from others
Move closer to those with whom they are talking
Initiate "social" touching behavior

supplies, other staff members are expected to cooperate because it is part of the assistant's job. The state inspector who examines radiographic equipment makes requests without fear of being ignored.

Expertise

Expertise means skill in performing valued services. The extensive training that dentists receive constitutes one basis for patients' and staff's deferring to them on dental matters. The hygienists' training is also a relative basis of power. Office managers can often build an independent power base on financial and management skills. Anyone in the office can become powerful if his or her job grows so complex that no one else can understand it.

Having Something Desirable

There are many rewards a dentist can dispense or withhold from staff: salaries and fringe benefits, working hours and conditions, and assignment of tasks, to name a few. Patients may respect dentists' status and expertise, but they probably come to the office most often because dentists can give them something they need—relief from pain and uncertainty and improved function and aesthetics.

The power to influence others' behavior using desired things tends to evaporate as soon as needs are satisfied. It is why the dentist and employees tend to behave differently before a new auxiliary is hired and after the probationary period. It also helps explain why patients are so compliant in the dental office and seem to disregard advice as soon as they leave.

Communication Skills Enhance Power

Being entitled to power is not the same thing as using it effectively. Communication skills multiply interpersonal influence, which derives from position, expertise, and having things that are desired. Without the kinds of skills taught throughout this book, these natural bases of power may be wasted.

Balance of Power in the Dental Office

In theory the dental office is a power hierarchy with the staff deferring to the dentist and the patient deferring to everyone. In reality, it is a complex and shifting network of relationships governed by different power balances. The assistant has the position or the delegated authority to order new supplies. The dealer's representative has the power of expertise based on knowledge of new products. The dentist has what both of them want, the power of agreement to buy. Whose views will prevail often depends on who is most persuasive. The hygienist brings position and expertise to bear in suggesting that the patient have bite-wing radiographs taken. The patient negotiates from the position of possessing power to give the needed assent. In some offices, the most powerful person may be an assistant whose understanding of human nature, command of language, and personal charm outweigh the primary power bases of others in the office.

CHAUVINISM

Chauvinism means consciously or unconsciously using language to manipulate others' status and erode their natural power.[3] This is in opposition to respect, which is expressing a credible belief in others' power. Respect is shown by a hygienist who treats a teenaged patient as a mature adult during diet counseling. When communication becomes barely credible and elevates anothers' status for ulterior motives, it is called flattery.

In this section we examine some of the ways in which chauvinism is expressed through depersonalization and presumption, and how it is particularly directed at women and people whose speech is different.

Depersonalization and Presumption

A common form of chauvinism works by dehumanizing the listener or the person spoken about.[4] "All kids are behavior problems" or "all auxiliaries are immature and should be called 'girls' " are examples of depersonalizing stereotypes that remove the speaker from having to relate to individuals on a personal basis. Sometimes this is expressed nonverbally through lack of eye contact, blank stares, or a deadpan tone of voice. Some dentists and auxiliaries discuss patients in their presence as if they did not exist.

The damage caused by depersonalization can be illustrated by the true story of a French soldier who fought for Napoleon and openly expressed his devotion to the war effort and love of his country. In a 1831 play, this man's political zeal was characterized and exaggerated. In time the character became more important than the play and his name was distorted into an epithet for blind and exaggerated self-pride. This was an unjust depersonalization and gross exaggeration of the soldier—what we now call chauvinism. But that is what this chapter is about—the damaging misconceptions we harbor about those we choose not to know as individuals. The soldier's name was Nicholas Chauvin.

Presumptive behavior, which seemingly denies listeners any choice, also communicates chauvinism. A list of twelve presumptive and destructive remarks is shown in Table 4–2.

Women as Victims

There is ample evidence that women in America are more likely than men to be the victims of chauvinism.[6,7] Table 4–3 displays some of the common differences in the way men and women speak and are spoken to. Sex also plays a role in perceived credibility. An example is seen in the often replicated study[8] in which college students read a passage that presents a persuasive message. The message is attributed to either John T. McKay or Joan T. McKay. Although the message is the same, students find John McKay more convincing than Joan. All subjects in the original study were

TABLE 4–2. TWELVE PRESUMPTIVE REMARKS THAT HAVE CHAUVINISTIC EFFECTS[5]

Type of Remark	Example
1. Ordering, directing, demanding	"You really should try. I expect it of you."
2. Warning, threatening	"You'd better keep at it or else."
3. Moralizing, preaching	"Oh, Mrs. Butterfield, I'm sure you want the best care possible."
4. Advising, giving solutions	"If you don't have time to floss at night, try arranging a few minutes at work."
5. Lecturing, teaching, giving facts	"Up to 90% of tooth loss could be prevented by . . ."
6. Judging, blaming, criticizing	"I really don't think you're trying."
7. Praising, buttering up	"You seem like you could do anything if you set your mind to it."
8. Name-calling, ridiculing	"I call patients like you 'dental cripples.'"
9. Interpreting, analyzing	"You just don't appreciate the value of this approach right now."
10. Reassuring, sympathizing	"I know how you feel, but everything will be okay."
11. Probing, questioning, interrogating	"But why don't you try this?"
12. Withdrawing, diverting, distracting	"Well, let's not talk about that now."

TABLE 4–3. EXAMPLES OF LANGUAGE DIFFERENCES BETWEEN MEN AND WOMEN.[7]

Women are more apt to . . .

Ways of Speaking	Ways of Being Spoken to
Speak better English	Receive flattery and false compliments
Use more emotion words	Hear euphemisms—polite words for "unmentionable" topics
Avoid taboos such as sex and rough language	Be called by first name
Use more intensifiers such as "very" and "really"	Be touched
Giggle	Be referred to in diminutive or subordinate status such as "the wife" or "my girls"
Lower eyes while talking	
Use qualifiers such as "I'm not sure, but" or "I kinda think . . ."	

women. It is quite possible that a male dentist would be perceived as more effective in presenting personal oral hygiene than a female hygienist even though both have comparable expertise and communication skills.

Those Whose Speech Differs

Chauvinism is often applied to children, the elderly, the poor, minority groups, foreigners, and others who talk differently. It is sometimes argued that black Americans are intellectually inferior because they persist in using nonstandard English as opposed to emigrant groups such as the Italians, Russians, or Polish who managed to erase all traces of accent within a few generations. Linguists have now discovered that blacks speak dialects that have sophisticated and internally consistent grammatical rules of their own.[9] There are also regional and ethnic differences among middle-class white speech, such as "might could," which is heard among the best educated in the Carolinas.

When giving descriptions, individuals from lower socioeconomic groups do tend to be more personal, concrete, and disorganized.[10] It may thus require more time to elicit a complete and accurate history from a patient who skips around and has difficulty relating to the dentist's perspective.

CONSEQUENCES OF CHAUVINISM AND RESPECT

The effects of damaging and unhealthy manipulations of others' status are predictable. Chauvinists have cultivated a "blindness" to this negative feedback, but they still must pay the price.

Apathy and Communication Breakdown

People who undermine the integrity of others by the way they talk elevate their own status at the cost of poor communication and strained interpersonal relations.[11] A domineering front desk staff member may keep all the auxiliaries in a subordinate position and may herd patients around efficiently. This staff member will get power and status, but the other auxiliaries and even the dentist will avoid the front desk, information will no longer pass through this important center, and cooperation will be reluctant. In the worst case, staff and patients will leave the practice. The telltale signs are nonverbal: slow responses, lack of eye contact, unbelieving stares, avoidance, and confusion.

Chauvinism, particulary if repeated, results in apathy—victims turn off their emotions; they stop caring. This creates new communication barriers. Victims of chauvinism are disinterested and lack normal emotion and attention. As a protective mechanism, they may have developed habits of distorting what they hear. Typically, they seek to avoid all communication with the chauvinist. Anger is a less common reaction, and one that actually signals that attempts at chauvinism are ineffective.

The apathy and the poor communication that chauvinism creates make the condition exceedingly difficult to reverse. It is usually a self-reinforcing downward spiral. The more the victim withdraws and hides his or her feelings, the more the chauvinist feels justified in depersonalizing the victim.

The following examples show how destructive linguistic chauvinism can be in a dental practice.

- *(Dentist to assistant who appears upset at being told that she cannot have a raise)* "Oh, come on, it can't be that bad. That's just a typical female overreaction and I know when you think about it rationally, you'll see that I am right." (Likely consequences: assistant will keep her feelings to herself, future requests will more likely be ultimatums, dentist's judgment may no longer be accepted unquestioningly, assistant's work will suffer, communication and cooperation will decrease, dentist will no longer be sought for advice, and assistant may look for another job.)

- *(Receptionist to patient who arrives late for appointment)* "What are we going to do with you, Mr. Sanchez? A grown man like you should be able to keep track of time." (Likely consequences: patient will be angry and will give less complete and truthful answers on medical, dental, and insurance questions; may not elect ideal treatment plan; more likely will dispute bill or be delinquent in payment; and more likely will be late in the future as a result of natural avoidance of unpleasant situations.)

Positive Effects of Respect

Management science has clearly shown that one of the keys to motivation is communicated respect.[12] Co-workers and patients respond with rapport and improved performance if they perceive that they are accorded the status they think they are due. This is also the foundation on which good communication is based because defensive barriers are thus lowered. It has been observed that the best hearing aid is a realistic compliment.

STATUS BUILDING

How we reflect our status relations through speech grows out of long-standing habits. There are, however, three suggestions that can be offered for improving skill performance in this area.

Be Sensitive

It would be quixotic to embark on a crusade to eradicate all traces of chauvinism from our own or from others' communication. What we do urge is that much practice be exercised in identifying instances and manners of chauvinism and its consequences. This sensitivity should be combined with insight into needs and values. Such awareness helps solve many interpersonal problems that otherwise remain enigmatic.

Be Assertive

When you are the victim of unfair status manipulations, the response of choice is assertiveness. Assertiveness is also a sound alternative for those tending to be chauvinistic. The next chapter is devoted to this skill. Consciously choosing to communicate respect likewise diminishes chauvinism.

Be Conservative

When in doubt about how much status to give a person, it is prudent to err in the direction of being too formal. The new patient, Mrs. Klosterman, will enjoy telling you that you may call her Betsy. The patient who thinks of herself as Mrs. O'Shea will take offense at being called Ms. O'Shea. Informality is not the same as respect and caring. When staff members have agreed to function on a first-name basis, they must still take care to observe expected formalities in the presence of patients to avoid causing confusion between informality and lack of professionalism.

CASE: POWERING OUT OF A TIGHT SPOT

The dentist showed the insurance salesman into his private office and motioned to a chair for the visitor to sit in. "Gee, it's nice of you to come out. I really appreciate your fitting it in to my busy schedule. It's been all catch up since I got back from London. Have you ever been to London, Jim?"

The agent sat and look up, "Well, actually, Dr. Barker, I was there during the war. Really, I was stationed in Plymouth, but we got up there several times..."

As the salesman spoke, the dentist walked around behind his desk, "You wouldn't recognize it now." He leaned forward gesturing as if to put his hand on the agent's arm. "And the prices! You wouldn't believe it. Dinner for two—$125. This sweater here cost $80." He sat back in his swivel chair and repeated, "$80. But tell me, how's business?"

The agent spoke briefly and generally about the American economy. The dentist looked at his guest for a minute then let his gaze wander out the window behind him.

This general conversation continued for some time with the dentist interrupting on occasion to change topics or interject his feelings. Finally, the salesman looked down at his briefcase and announced, half apologetically and half hopefully, "Well, there's some things I'd like to show you if you don't mind."

ANALYSIS

At first it may appear that the dentist is just wasting time socializing and being a little pompous. On closer inspection it can be seen that he is shrewdly manipulating power to his advantage.

The dentist calls his visitor by first name, which is either a sign of intimacy or of superior status in the speaker.[13] The agent is forced to acknowledge the dentist's title by calling him Dr. Barker, thereby accepting the lower status position. The gestures and movement in the room as well as control over topics belong to the dentist. He indicates through interruptions and poor eye contact that the salesman has unimportant things to say. In fact, the dentist never acknowledges the reason for the visit. Talking about money and speaking in very concrete terms also shows the dentist's power.

It is unlikely that the dentist is just being boorish, even if this behavior is unconscious. Putting the salesman in a "one-down" position makes it easier for the dentist to save time in declining to buy insurance or may pay off in more attractive terms if he decides to buy. Caution: This game must be played carefully and subtly. Most good salesmen are experts.

REFERENCES

1. Scott, M.D., & Powers, W.G. *Interpersonal communication: A question of needs.* Boston: Houghton Mifflin, 1978.
2. French, J.R.P., Jr., & Raven, B. The bases of social power. In D. Cartwright (Ed.), *Studies in social power.* Ann Arbor: University of Michigan Institute of Social Research, 1959, pp. 150–167.
3. Satir, R. *Peoplemaking.* Palo Alto: Science and Behavior Books, 1972.
4. Hall, E.T. *The silent language.* Greenwich, Conn.: Fawcett, 1959.
5. Gordon, T. *P.E.T. in action.* New York: Bantam Books, 1976.
6. Chafetz, J.S. *Masculine/feminine or human? An overview of the sociology of sex roles.* Itasca, Ill.: F. E. Peacock Publishers, 1974.
7. Shostrom, E.L., & Kavanaugh, J. *Between man and woman.* Los Angeles: Nash Publishing, 1971.
8. Key, M.R. Linguistic behavior of male and female. *Linguistics,* 1972, 88, 15–31.
9. Dillard, J.L. *Black English.* New York: Random House, 1972.
10. Schatzman, L., & Strauss, A.L. Social class and mode of communication. *American Journal of Sociology,* 1955, 60, 329–338.
11. Blau, P.M. *Exchange and power in social life.* New York: Wiley, 1964.
12. Whetten, D.A., & Cameron, K.S. *Developing management skills.* Glenview, Ill.: Scott, Foresman and Company, 1984.
13. Brown, R., & Gilman, A. The pronouns of power and solidarity. In T.A. Sebeok (Ed.), *Style in Language.* Cambridge: MIT Press, 1960, pp. 253–276.

EXERCISES

4–1. Select a television drama or movie you have not seen before. Watch a few minutes with the sound off. See if you can tell who has the dominant status in each group based solely on nonverbal communication. Make a list of the clues that indicate status. Turn up the sound to confirm your prediction. What additional verbal cues do you notice?

4–2. Select a one-time interaction with a stranger, such as a waiter, tour guide, clerk, or bureaucrat. Status in this situation is usually undetermined in advance. Use Table 4-1 as a guide and practice either dominant or submissive communication behavior. Use this behavior when meeting or telephoning such a person for the first time. Pay particular attention to the status communications you receive back. As a variation, you may experiment with a friend who has a different status (teacher, employee, parent). Practice sending inappropriate status messages and observe both your own and your friend's reactions.

4–3. Select a date when you want to observe the effects of personal power. On a piece of paper or large note card write the date at the top and make four columns: "behavior," "initiator," "basis," and "resistance." During the day write down examples of behavior that you would not normally engage in were it not for someone else's power. Also note the name of the person who initiated your behavior. At the end of the day, indicate the basis of each power action: position, expertise, something desired, or communication skill. Also note anything you did or could have done to resist or reduce the initiator's power. As a variation, you may wish to substitute "receiver" for the "initiator" heading and take your own power inventory by recording the behavior you cause others to undertake.

4–4. Puncture some stereotypes. Before dealing with a colleague or acquaintance, such as a classmate, a spouse, or a patient, take a minute to learn something new and personal about them. Use the conversation skills described in Chapter 3. Observe the effect on your normal interaction with that person.

4–5. Review your notes for Exercise 4–3. In your list of power relations, can you identify anywhere you feel the relationship involved unnatural and destructive status differences? How is the linguistic chauvinism expressed? What is the effect on the victim?

DISCUSSION OF EXERCISES

4–1. Table 4–1 contains many nonverbal communication patterns typical of status interactions. There may be obvious signs such as dress, office or room arrangement, and other status symbols. If the segment you are watching involves conversation among very close friends, you will likely notice less status communication. In special circumstances, such as asking favors, status communication can be distorted or exaggerated. Repeat the exercise several times and notice how much more sensitive you become to this dimension of communication.

4–2. You should find that the stranger very quickly adopts a *complimentary* style of status communication. After the pattern has been established, try to switch your status. You will observe either confusion or resistance. This shows how quickly status relationships are developed. The exercise with a friend of higher or lower status shows that status and intimacy are separate and not inconsistent dimensions of human relations.

4–3. Most people who interact with others and are consciously recording cannot complete even part of a day. It is surprising how much of your behavior is controlled by others' power. Status and having something are the most frequently reported power bases and avoidance is used most often to screen against unwanted power interactions.

4–4. A stereotype is a generalization which prevents treating another person as an individual by depersonalizing him or her. Stereotypes may be very strong for people you have known a long time. Individualizing others as the first stage of any interaction usually promotes good rapport and trust. You should also observe more spontaneous communication.

4–5. Compare your list with others and you will likely find that there are differences in whether status interactions are perceived as natural and beneficial or artificial and detrimental.

5

Assertiveness

Assertiveness means expressing your rights or doing your job without insisting that you get your own way by manipulating others. Telling a companion or a stranger that their smoking bothers you or reminding an employee of the need to be punctual are examples of assertive communication.

The three sections in this chapter each answer a question: When is it appropriate to be assertive? How should assertiveness be communicated? Must one always be assertive?

WHEN IS IT APPROPRIATE TO BE ASSERTIVE?

An assertive response is appropriate when another's behavior is causing a problem, provided that we have a legal or professional responsibility, or when our own rights are being threatened. The dentist can be assertive about a receptionist who is rude to patients (job responsibility) but not about the kind of car the receptionist drives. The assistant can be assertive when the dentist makes chauvinistic remarks (personal rights threatened) but not when new charting procedures are instituted. The rules for making nonassertive suggestions are discussed below.

Those Who Own Problems May be Assertive

Any unmet need is a problem. A patient who is chatting with the receptionist to pass the time while waiting to see the dentist has no problem. But the receptionist who needs to catch up on billing has a time problem. A patient who needs privacy is embarrassed by the inadvisable practice of having to discuss financial matters at the front desk, within earshot of other patients. Those whose needs are not met are said to "own the problem."[1]

Being careful to solve only our own problems helps prevent interpersonal conflicts. Consider the dentist who cannot tolerate inefficiency, personally or in others. Advice given to the receptionist who is getting good results through extra effort is most likely to generate resentment. When a patient expresses lack of confidence in a hygienist who looks young, the hygienist's problem is establishing trust, not straightening out the patient's hang-ups. The first step in being assertive is to recognize which problems are ours and to avoid trying to solve those of others.

RESPONSIBILITIES LEAD TO ASSERTIVENESS. It is appropriate to be assertive when the problems we own adversely affect areas for which we are responsible. Health professionals are responsible for the care, safety, and dignity of patients. Dentists may delegate authority for various aspects of care to staff members, but ultimate responsibility remains with the dentist. Hence the dentist is justifiably concerned and "owns every problem" resulting from staff behavior that affects any aspect of patient care.

Professionals may not always welcome the problems they own as a result of their responsibilities, but it is part of professionalism to address such problems as the ones mentioned below before they seriously affect patient care.

- Dentist speaks to the assistant about errors in ordering supplies (office efficiency affects patient care and is thus ultimately the dentist's responsibility).
- Assistant restrains child who is squirming in the chair (to protect patient and operator).
- Dentist obtains complete and accurate medical history (to protect patient and reduce opportunity for lawsuit in the event of mishap).

INTERPERSONAL RIGHTS LEAD TO ASSERTIVENESS. It is appropriate to be assertive when the problem we own is a threat to our rights. Dentists, staff, and patients alike are entitled to the rights shown in Table 5–1. When these rights are challenged, as when a patient verbally abuses the receptionist or when the den-

TABLE 5–1. COMMON RIGHTS IN INTERPERSONAL RELATIONS

Right	Example of Threat or Violation
One's own feelings	"You should be glad it's not worse." "Its silly to cry over such a small thing."
Freedom of action (provided we accept consequences)	"You don't have any choice in the matter."
Freedom from self-justification	"What do you mean, 'you don't know'?" "How can you refuse my request?"
Speak up for own rights	"I don't want to hear about your problems." "My decision is nonnegotiable."

tist establishes new nonnegotiable office hours without consulting the staff, an assertive response is in order.[2,3]

BEING ASSERTIVE VERSUS GIVING ADVICE. Regardless of how strongly one feels the need to help others or share insight, when problems do not stem from our responsibilities or rights, we are unjustified in being assertive. Instead we may give advice. Giving advice requires that two conditions be met: (1) rapport must exist and (2) permission must be received.[4] Even among friends there are times when one is too tense, tired, or preoccupied to want to listen to the best of suggestions.

The following examples illustrate problems that do not involve responsibility or rights, but where permission is being asked to give advice.

- *(One co-worker to another)* "I noticed that Mr. Bluster was giving you a hard time, too. Do you want to hear how I learned to handle outbursts like that?"
- *(Hygienist to patient)* "I think we are good enough friends for me to speak freely about some of the problems you are having brushing. Would you like to hear about some new techniques that might help?"
- *(Anyone to anyone else)* "You look worried. Is it anything I can help with?"

COMMUNICATING ASSERTIVELY

Interpersonal conflict always involves more than one person, so satisfactory solutions are never entirely under one person's control. Although there are no guaranteed successful techniques, there are some strategies that maximize the opportunity for success. When our responsibilities and our rights impel us to be assertive, we want to express real issues clearly, state who "owns the problem," and minimize defensiveness.

Three techniques—"solution suggestion," "I-messages," and "DESC scripts"—can be used to communicate assertiveness (Table 5–2). Solution suggestion is for spontaneous responses to problems of no great importance. DESC scripts are appropriate when the problem is momentous or long-standing, and they require advanced preparation. I-messages occupy a middle position.

Solution Suggestion

The easiest type of assertive response specifies the behavior one wants while ignoring issues of blame.[3] It is effective when the problem is caused by another's oversight or carelessness or for matters too small to deserve a formal response.

- *(Dentist to patient)* "I would appreciate your not moving around in the chair."

TABLE 5–2. THREE TECHNIQUES FOR ASSERTIVENESS

Situation: A staff meeting degenerates into name calling.

Message	Example
Suggested solution	
Specify desired behavior	"Let's focus on the dental problem, not on finding blame."
I–message	
Describe problem behavior	"When we get into personalities . . ."
Express how speaker feels	"I get upset . . ."
Tangible effects of problem	". . . because this is eroding everybody's morale."
DESC script	
Describe problem behavior	"When we get into personalities . . ."
Express how speaker feels	"I get upset."
Specify desired behavior	"Let's focus on the dental problem, not on finding blame."
Consequences	"I'm sure this will be more productive." (or) ". . . otherwise I'm going to call this meeting to a halt and decide this myself."

- *(Dentist to assistant)* "Let's get this lab tidied up."
- *(Hygienist to patient whose conversation is too personal)* "Now we have to concentrate on the dental problem here."

I-Messages

I-messages, which are useful in more serious situations, are statements that let others know how their behavior is causing problems.[3] There are three parts to a well-constructed I-message: (1) a description of what others are doing that causes a problem (the cause), (2) an expression of how the speaker feels (the problem), and (3) identification of the tangible effects (the result). The order of the three components can be varied and the tangible effects may be left unspoken. But tangible effects must exist; otherwise assertiveness would not be appropriate.

- *(Dentist to patient)* "I'm disappointed that you want the extraction rather than letting me save the tooth. I am afraid you will not think I have given you the best care possible."
- *(Staff to dentist)* "When you refer to us as 'the girls' it demoralizes me because I feel unprofessional."
- *(Chairside assistant to dentist)* "When you are in a hurry and reach for instruments yourself it makes me nervous because I lose the sequence of the routine and I am less help to you."
- *(Dentist to patient)* "When you come late, you put me in a tight spot. I dislike having to remind you of your responsibility and I am late with my other patients."

The power of I-messages comes from the speaker sharing his or her problem in an unarguable fashion. When the hygienist says, "I am disappointed by your homecare efforts," the patient cannot contradict, "Oh, no you're not" or complain, "I don't know why you are upset."

The effectiveness of I-messages is compromised when the problem behavior is exaggerated ("you're always late") or when it is too general ("you're so ineffective"). Another common error is to disguise a judgmental remark in an apparent I-statement ("I think you are uninformed" or "I find you offensive").

DESC Scripts

DESC scripts (pronounced desk) are reserved for important and typically recurring problems such as the obnoxious patient, the habitual put-down, or the chronically late employee.[2] DESC is an acronymn for (1) *describing* the problem behavior, (2) *expressing* feelings, (3) *specifying* desired alternatives, and (4) identifying *consequences*. Table 5–2 shows that DESC scripts contain the first two statements in an I-message, followed by a solution suggestion. The fourth part of a DESC script, the consequences, is the speaker's promise to do something based on how others respond to the suggested solution. A full DESC script sounds like this.

- *(Dentist to chairside assistant)* "When you and the other staff smile and look at each other in staff meetings but don't say anything (describe), I feel frustrated and sometimes annoyed (express). It would be more helpful to me if you let me know what is on your mind (specify). I promise to listen openly if you will only speak up, otherwise it puts a strain on our whole relationship (consequences)."
- *(Assistant to dentist)* "I have asked several times in the past weeks for a reconsideration of my raise. Each time you say you're too busy (describe) and I feel put-down (express). I think you're busy now, but I know you have some time tomorrow at 4:30 and I would like to talk then (specify). I want to continue working for someone who values my contribution but I can't perform well when I'm not part of the team (consequences)."

The addition of consequences, either positive or negative, makes DESC scripts effective. First, they show that the speaker has thought through the problem and, second, they signal that the listener now has a problem. This forms the basis for negotiation and the person who has analyzed the range of desired behaviors and appropriate consequences is in the strongest bargaining position. DESC scripts are difficult to deliver extemporaneously. Time is required to weigh alternative behaviors and consequences and to rehearse an effective presentation.

MUST ONE ALWAYS BE ASSERTIVE?

The alternatives to assertiveness are aggression and acquiescence.[5] Aggressive people try to manipulate others, to gain status at others' expense, and to ignore others' rights. Aggresive behavior need not be loud and threatening. A dentist who refuses to discuss salaries is aggressive because the staff member's right to a hearing is denied. A hygienist who uses "feminine wiles" to get special privileges is equally aggressive.

Acquiescence means temporarily surrendering one's rights because greater needs exist. The dentist may smile at the patient and say, "No, I don't mind going over plaque control again," when the dentist is actually thinking, "this is the hygienist's job and I am two patients behind." In this case it is the dentist's feelings and behaviors that are being compromised. Some examples of assertive, aggressive, and acquiescent communication are listed below.

- The dentist is running late at the end of the day and has several errands to do before a six o'clock meeting. The receptionist appears in the operatory door and says, "It's Dr. Bertolli again. He needs more information on that referral."
  a. "Would you tell him it would be difficult for me to leave my patient now and ask if I can return his call about nine tomorrow?" (Assertion)
  b. Can't you see I'm in the middle of something? Tell him I'll call him when I can." (Aggression)
  c. "Okay." (Acquiescence)
- The hygienist finds the operatory sloppy and disorganized each morning and the assistant who is supposed to clean this area is uncooperative. The hygienist takes the problem to the dentist.
  a. "I am having to do part of another person's job and when an instrument I need isn't clean I lose time and the patient's confidence. This makes me feel less professional and also a little used." (Assertion)
  b. "Why don't you make that new assistant do the job right?" (Aggression)
  c. "I guess you want me to police my own area." (Acquiescence)

Reasons for Acquiescence

Of the two alternatives to assertiveness, acquiescence is more common in dental settings. Dental professionals are typically under time pressure, they are uncomfortable with emotions, and they are supposed to "serve" patients. Table 5–3 lists some of the reasons why a person might choose to temporarily suspend the right to be assertive. Most of these reasons are sound at times and in certain contexts. It is therefore clear that the habit of always being assertive is unnatural and unwise.

Costs of Acquiescence

Even though acquiescence may be an appropriate alternative to assertiveness, there are costs associated with it. Temporarily sub-

TABLE 5–3. REASONS FOR BEING ACQUIESCENT

Reason	Rationale
Loss of power	"I will show how big I am by not 'coming down' on everyone who deserves it."
Fear of retaliation	"If I say something I'll have to pay for it later or it will damage our friendship."
Forfeit protective habits	"I'm the loyal type who doesn't make waves." (or) "My co-workers are too unreasonable to try to explain myself."
Fear loss of emotional control	"I'm afraid of what I might say." (or) "We shouldn't talk about feelings."
Abused helper	"A professional is a public servant. The customer is always right."
Time and energy	"I'm too busy to deal with it now. It's not worth the effort."
Assertiveness is a learned skill	"Aggression is my only alternative. I don't know how to express my rights without being offensive."

ordinating interpersonal rights or responsibilities to more pressing needs builds up a backlog of unresolved problems and guilt. A history of acquiescence often precedes an aggressive overreaction in which frustrations are displaced onto an innocent third party. Patients are sometimes made to bear the burden of unresolved staff tension. Even spouses and friends pay for our decision not to face up to a patient who is abusive. A dangerous result of repeated long-term acquiescence is developing an "acquiescent personality." When giving up our rights and responsibilities becomes an habitual response, we are compromised as professionals and as people. Finally, acquiescence adversely affects communication because acquiescent messages tend to be ambiguous. When a dentist accepts a referral patient against his or her better judgment, the mumbled response, "What's one more problem in my life of endless problems?" leaves the referring dentist with doubts about what has been said.

A Strategy for Assertiveness

All of us can become more assertive. We can manage our problems in a constructive fashion and suggest solutions, use I-messages, and deliver DESC scripts to negotiate for more fulfilling relationships. Those who would like to work on developing assertive skills might review the four steps in the following plan.

ANALYZE THE PROBLEM. It is profitable to spend some time identifying the circumstances in which assertiveness is needed. Patterns usually exist concerning certain types of individuals, topics, and environments or times when we feel pressured, threatened, or fatigued. It is our right to choose situations in which we want to be assertive and in which the probable rewards do not justify the effort. A good way to begin is to select a mildly threatening, but predictably recurring situation, such as with a patient or co-worker with an irritating mannerism. Small initial successes supply the self-esteem and tactics needed for larger problems.

PREPARE. Until assertiveness becomes habitual, we must plan before speaking up for our rights and responsibilities. DESC scripts can be written and rehearsed, alone or with friends, before they are actually delivered. It is also useful to anticipate the variety of reactions that others might exihibit when you become assertive.

ANALYZE THE RESULTS. Assertive behavior will only develop into a habit when it becomes rewarding. Success will result in more satisfying relations with others who change their behavior because they respect our rights. Another reward is a change in the way we feel. Most acquiescent individuals who speak assertively are surprised at their sense of self-satisfaction and pride. Even when no behavior is changed, they need no longer feel guilty or apologetic. For assertive behavior, a small notebook or three by five cards with the headings "setting," "situation," "my behavior," "results," and "my feelings" can provide useful insight if kept for several months.

READ AND ATTEND WORKSHOPS. Seminars and self-help groups can be located through community colleges and service organization. Many books are available.[2,3,6–8]

CASE: HOW FEET GRAVITATE TOWARD THE MOUTH

In the case that follows the dentist speaks to the hygienist about a problem and the hygienist discusses a problem with her roommate. Neither situation is well handled. Before reading the analysis at the end of the case, try to decide who owns each problem, what responsibilities and rights are involved, whether intervention is required or optional in each situation, and what Bill Meyers and Janice Pudwell should have said.

The last patient of the day had just left the operatory and Janice Pudwell was hurriedly putting away her instruments. The dentist appeared at the door, leaning on the edge of the counter with his hands on his hips, and said, "Janice, I think we had better have a little talk."

The hygienist answered, "Okay," with a slight tone of defeat and sat down on her stool facing the autoclave, still holding instruments in each hand.

"You've really been flubbing up all week. That last patient had pretty pronounced trauma on the buccal of the molars. You seem to be rushing your work. And I hear you raised your voice to Grace yesterday. There's just no excuse for this kind of behavior. I won't tolerate it in my office. What is going on, anyway?"

"Oh, nothing, really," the hygienist answered. "I'm sorry if I've upset you." She resumed sorting the instruments.

Bill Meyers folded his arms across his chest and leaned against the counter. "You know, this isn't like you. You've been acting strange."

Janice looked directly at the dentist for the first time and said, "Well, it's nothing to do with the office. It's personal and I don't feel like talking about it. It doesn't really concern anyone here." She looked down at her hands again.

"Oh, okay then," answered the dentist. "I make it a rule not to interfere in the personal lives of my staff. I would be glad to listen sometime if you think I could help. Okay? Well, I have to get back to my patient . . ."

The hygienist waited just long enough for the dentist to enter his operatory, then hurried to the front desk and made a phone call.

"Hi, Pat, it's me. . . . I'm sorry to keep bothering you but what did he say? Did you get your job back? . . . Well, since I am the one who suggested that you come right out and tell him what you think of the way he treated you, I think I have a right to be concerned. Maybe it wasn't any of my business, but it's just not fair how he takes advantage of everybody. . . . We should stand up for our rights . . ."

ANALYSIS

The dentist has a problem. A normally pleasant and efficient hygienst is not treating patients in a satisfactory manner and is causing friction in the office. This is a situation that requires a response, but the global and accusing remarks he makes prompt a defensive response from the hygienist. Personal problems cease to be private when they interfere with patient care or staff morale. An assertive remark is needed at this point: "I have no intention of prying into your personal affairs, but your treatment of the past patient and of Grace has me upset. I will be in an hour early tomorrow and I would like to see you then so we can work this out. I don't like to see a valuable employee let the office down without knowing why."

The hygienist's roommate, Pat, also has a problem. She has been urged to take an assertive stand with her employer. Janice Pudwell is trying to take over her roommate's problem. This situation involves giving advice and rather than pushing in with repeated apologies, Janice might have said, "I've been thinking about you all day. Can you talk about it?"

REFERENCES

1. Gordon, T.E. *P.E.T. in action.* New York: Bantam Books, 1976.
2. Bower, S.A., and Bower, G.H. *Asserting yourself: A practical guide for positive change.* Reading, Mass.: Addison-Wesley, 1976.
3. Clark, C.C. *Assertive skills for nurses.* Wakefield, Mass.: Contemporary Publishing, 1978.
4. Morton, J.C., & Blair, D. Encouraging others to change their behavior. In J.E. Jones & J.W. Pfeiffer (eds.), *1979 Handbook for group facilitators.* La Jolla, Calif.: University Associates, 1979.
5. Smith, M.J. *When I say no, I feel guilty.* New York: Dial Books, 1975.
6. Alberti, R.E., & Emmons, M.L. *Your perfect rights* (rev. ed.). San Luis Obispo, Calif.: Impact Press, 1974.
7. Galassi, M.D., & Gallasi, J.P. *Assert yourself: How to be your own person.* New York: Human Sciences Press, 1977.
8. Osborn, S., & Harris, G. *Assertive training for women.* Springfield, Ill.: Charles C. Thomas, 1975.

EXERCISES

5–1. For each of the following situations, identify who owns the problem and what need is unmet.

a. The dentist mutters, "I can't read the receptionist's handwriting. I'm going to have to do something about this."

b. The receptionist says to a patient, "Excuse me, Mr. Doyle, you have an outstanding balance which is getting rather large."

c. The patient listens to the case presentation and then responds, "I know you just want what is best for me, but I don't really want to spend $1300 right now and you said that the last option with the extractions would work okay, right?"

5–2. Decide whether each of the cases below requires a response, permits giving advice, or neither. Identify the rights or responsibilities involved.

a. The dentist overhears the receptionist and the patient arguing.

b. A new patient declines to answer the question on the registration form about previous dentists.

c. A patient of many years seems unusually terse and defensive.

5–3. Determine whether each of the following behaviors is assertive, aggressive, or acquiescent.

a. After the patient declines the "optimal" treatment plan, the dentist answers, "Well, I don't want to tell you what to do, but my professional opinion is that you are making a big mistake and you will regret that choice."

b. A dentist tells the hygienist, "You've put me in an awkward position with Mr. France by suggesting that his bridge will have to be replaced."

c. Dentist in staff meeting, "I might as well save my breath. Nothing I say about keeping the lab neat seems to have any effect."

5–4. For the two situations below, write a solution suggestion, an I-message, and a DESC script.

a. A patient talks constantly while in the chair, preventing you from proceeding with treatment.

b. A patient or co-worker is smoking in the reception area, despite posted signs requesting no smoking.

DISCUSSION OF EXERCISES

5–1. a. The dentist owns this problem because of unmet needs for information, lost time in clarification, and perhaps threatened sense of control. The receptionist will not have a problem until the dentist says something.

b. Needing to discharge job responsibilities is the source of the receptionist's problem.

c. Both the dentist and the patient have problems. The patient needs to make a choice between optimal care and limited financial resources, or perhaps fear of more extensive procedures. Dentists are seldom disinterested observers in such situations. They have feelings about ideal and unacceptable treatments, they care about their patients, and their ego as a persuader may be on the line.

5–2. a. Arguments will erode staff morale and alienate patients, and both have adverse affects on patient care. Because the dentist is responsible for all aspects of patient care, this situation requires an assertive response.

b. No intervention is appropriate initially because care is unlikely to be affected. Once rapport has been established, the subject can be broached.

c. A dental professional may offer advice because rapport exists, provided that permission is asked. Patients have the right not to explain their feelings.

5–3. a. The unequal status of professional and patient and the persistence in pressing for the dentist's choice make this case an example of aggression.

b. The dentist asserts feelings of compromised authority without attacking the hygienist in this example of assertion.

c. The dentist is acquiescing by making a joke and acknowledging a practice that is unacceptable.

5–4. a. "Please be quiet while I complete this examination." "I can't get your work done when you're talking and that makes me anxious." "Your constant talking upsets me. I would like you to remain quiet until I can finish this procedure. That will allow me to concentrate and do a better job. (If I get too distracted, I'll have to reappoint you to finish the procedure.)"

b. "Could you smoke outside, please?" "Your smoking bothers me because it irritates my eyes." "I am bothered by your smoking and would be grateful if you would observe the signs requesting that you don't. (Otherwise I will have to speak to the dentist.)"

6

Nonverbal Communication

Much of interpersonal communication is carried by facial expressions, gestures, pitch and pace of speech, eye contact, distance between speakers, dress, and touch. The exact blend varies from one situation to another, but one often-quoted estimate of the sources used for judging others' attitudes is 55 percent facial expression, 38 percent voice, and only 7 percent verbal content.[1]

The nonverbal aspects of communication are woven into most chapters of this text because they are part of *the way we communicate* and are seldom a substitute for written and spoken language. This chapter highlights the essential features of nonverbal communication. Once we have a common language to talk about the subject, nonverbal communication is applied to three situations in the dental context: reading patients, acting professionally, and touching.

CHARACTERISTICS OF NONVERBAL COMMUNICATION

Nonverbal communication is continuous, instantaneous, rich, subtle, and semiconscious.[2] Table 6–1 lists these five characteristics and their importance to dentistry.

Continuous

A perceptive observer can always learn something from facial expressions, posture, and mannerisms, even when nothing is being

TABLE 6–1. CHARACTERISTICS OF NONVERBAL COMMUNICATION

Characteristic	Importance in Dentistry
Continuous	Permits monitoring of patients and co-workers even when they are not talking
Instantaneous	Permits timely adjustments to others' feelings
Rich	Many sources of information available even when conversation is limited
Subtle	Precise shadings of feelings are possible even when patients lack vocabulary to describe them
Semiconscious	Nonverbals can usually be trusted

said in words. For example, patients who are reluctant to talk are expressing their discomfort, embarrassment, or fear without need of words.

Almost Instantaneous

Before an employee can object to what the dentist is saying, the employee's face and posture may already express a feeling. A skilled communicator can use this type of feedback to modify what is being said, even in midsentence.

Rich and Full

Words are one-dimensional and come out in single file. By contrast, the simultaneous, multidimensional picture created by posture, gestures, facial expression, tone, pitch, volume, and pace, to name a few sources, paint a vivid picture of the speaker.

Subtle

Most individuals are incapable of consistently choosing the precise term to express delicate shades of meaning. Length of pause and tentativeness of voice, on the other hand, can be adjusted to convey precisely the degree of skepticism or uncertainty desired.

Typically Semiconscious

Although we are occasionally aware of our voice or our posture, it is impossible to monitor consciously all aspects of verbal and nonverbal expression. The spontaneous quality of nonverbals is a source of their high credibility.

These features make nonverbal communication especially important in dentistry. The noise of the handpiece and the fact that patients characteristically have their mouths full of fingers and instruments mean that nonverbal communication is frequently the only practical method available. In dentistry the patient is vulnerable to physical pain and heightened emotions, and these may often be read in patients' faces. The teamwork required of the dentist and staff, particularly at chairside, makes nonverbal communication essential to a smooth practice. There simply is not enough time to say everything, and much that is communicated among professionals is best left unspoken in the patient's presence.

BODY LANGUAGE IS WHAT THE BODY SAYS

Known technically as kinesics, body language includes gestures, posture, facial expressions, and eye contact.[2] Body language can take the place of spoken communication, but more typically it accompanies and modifies verbal messages. Table 6–2 shows the four fundamental functions of nonverbal communication.[3]

In the following example, all four functions of body language are present. A receptionist draws little circles on the appointment pad and nods rhythmically as the patient explains why he needs an early morning appointment. Finally she raises her hand and shakes her head, "But I told you," she says, "the first appointment before nine is not until the 15th of the month." The raised hand is a universally understood signal to stop. The shaking head adds emphasis to what the receptionist is saying. Nodding while listening encourages the patient to speak. The doodling is a nervous characteristic that has no direct effect on communication.

TABLE 6–2. FOUR USES OF NONVERBAL COMMUNICATION

Use	Examples
Clear substitute for verbal communication	"V" sign for victory, horizontal outstretched arm with palm up for "stop," applause for approval
Gestures and facial expressions that amplify verbal message	Laughter, pointing, public speaking gestures, frowns
Expressions and gestures that control flow of communication	Head and eye movements to signal control, nodding agreement, level pitch and increasing volume to prevent interruption
Personal idiosyncrasies that accompany speech but have no meaning	Ritual with cigarettes, coffee cups, glasses; head and hand ticks; stammering

Nonverbals Substitute for Words

Gestures or facial movements such as the index finger to the lips or a hitchhiker's extended thumb are well enough understood to take the place of some verbal communication. The assistant indicates which operatory an adult patient is to use with an "after you" gesture of the arm. Young children are invited to come into the office by an outstretched hand. One of the roughly 70 gestures recognized by most Americans is the cheek in palm showing "I've got a toothache."[4]

Nonverbals Amplify Spoken Language

Patients point to their jaws and grimace when describing pain. The assistant shrugs a shoulder and looks puzzled when denying any knowledge of where the missing radiographs might be. On the other hand, discrepancies between the verbal and nonverbal aspects of communication are often a clue that something may be amiss in the spoken message.

Nonverbals Modify and Control the Way People Talk

Nodding and paying attention signal that the listener wants the speaker to continue. A steady pitch, slightly increased volume, and avoidance of eye contact characterize a speaker who does not want to be interrupted. Some of the ways nonverbal communication can control the way people talk are shown in Table 6–3.[5]

TABLE 6–3. HOW NONVERBAL COMMUNICATION REGULATES VERBAL COMMUNICATION

Turn Yielding—"Now you talk . . ."	Decreased volume, slower tempo, no gestures, relaxed posture, gazing at listener, "trailers" such as "you know" or "hum?", rising pitch at end of comment
Turn Maintaining—"No, I'm still talking . . ."	Increased volume and rate, filled pauses such as "er . . . er" or "I . . . I," few pauses and gestures to fill pauses, eye contact avoided
Turn Requesting—"I want to talk . . ."	Raised finger, audible inspiration of breath, straightening things, leaning forward, tense posture, interruption without eye contact and speaking loud and fast to avoid counterinterruption, fast and rhythmic head nodding and pretended or pseudoagreement
Turn Denying—"It's okay, you go on . . ."	Relaxed posture, no change in facial expression or eye contact, smiling, faciliation, silence

Some Nonverbals Are Unconscious and Insignificant Habits
Some of the habits associated with speaking are mistaken for meaningful nonverbal communication. Patients may bite their lips while talking to the dentist. This might mean that they are nervous and concerned about their mouth or it might be a natural habit signifying nothing at all. These habits are most significant when they change or stop. A dentist who hums while operating may scare patients by stopping the humming.

PARALANGUAGE IS THE WAY WE TALK

Paralanguage only occurs when we are talking, and then it is always present.[2] The principal elements are timing, pitch, volume, pace, voice quality, pauses, and nonfluencies such as "eh" and slips of the tongue. When the patient who agrees to follow a postoperative suggestion answers too quickly in a low voice, cutting off the end of words, some doubt can be raised about how genuine the agreement is.

There are circumstances in dentistry where the elements of paralanguage overshadow the verbal message. In the voice control technique used to break through children's crying and get their attention, it is the volume, firmness, and suddenness that matter and not what is said. Some dentists have experimented with semihypnotic, monotone, soft, repetitious language to relax patients. Tranquil paralanguage is important when patients are under nitrous oxide analgesia in order to minimize the risk of paradoxial reactions.

FINDING THE RIGHT DISTANCE

There are distances that are appropriate for certain relations between people and for certain activities.[6] Deviations from these socially expected distances cause tension and contribute to misunderstandings (Table 6–4).

Intimate Distance
At a distance of 0 to 18 inches individuals who are well known to each other express warmth and concern, and share private feelings and secrets. At this close range one's physical presence is overwhelming and it is impossible for the listener to pay attention to much else. Nonverbals are likely to overpower any verbal content in the message.

TABLE 6–4. INTERPERSONAL DISTANCE

Type	Distance	Relationship	Message
Intimate	1 to 18 inches	Intimates and very close friends	Confidence, intimacy
Personal	18 inches to 4 feet	Friends, equals	Personal information
Social	4 to 12 feet	Acquaintances	Conducting business
Public	12 feet or more	Strangers	Formal and status

Much of dentistry is performed at this intimate distance. Since no personal or emotional intimacy is intended, it is important that dentists, hygienists, and assistants be conscious of their professional manner. Jokes and personal remarks should be resisted when working in the patient's mouth. Posttreatment instructions and oral hygiene instruction given at this distance will be wasted because they are incongruous with patient's expectations for such settings.

Personal Distance

At a distance of a foot and a half to four feet interest in maintaining interpersonal relations is shown. This is the range at which dental professionals often talk to patients, usually pushing the stool back from the dental chair to present diagnostic findings or give instructions. The problem is that this may be uncomfortable for patients who are anxious or who do not feel "friendly." If patients were in chairs with wheels, it would not be uncommon to find them pushing even farther away from the dentist or hygienist when it came time to discuss serious business.

Social Distance

Most patients would prefer four to seven feet between them and the dentist when speaking. This is the distance the dentist would normally stand from the receptionist or other office staff while they are discussing the day's activities.

Public Distance

Distances over 12 feet express formality and status. Presidents of large corporations may have their desks situated so that no one can approach closer than 12 feet. Public distance in dentistry is rare and is discussed only in Chapter 19 on Speaking in Public.

Emotions Affect Personal Space

Every individual carries a personal space, typically two to four feet. Because dental professionals must constantly violate this space, they should be careful to observe the professional precautions of courtesy and formality when doing so.

Personality and mood can alter requirements for personal space.[7] Introverts tend to require more individual territory than their outgoing friends. Stress and anxiety increase the distance required as an interpersonal buffer. Some individuals will not tolerate closeness or being touched when they are angry, frightened, or tired. Professionals who are sensitive to the territorial needs of patients and co-workers who are under pressure can improve the effectiveness of their communication dramatically by adding a foot or two more distance.

READING PATIENTS' AND CO-WORKERS' NONVERBALS

Reading nonverbal communication follows the SIT principle: (1) place the gesture, expression, or voice characteristic in the total *s*ituation; (2) *i*nterpret its meaning tentatively, as an hypothesis, and (3) *t*est to verify that your interpretation is meaningful.

- **S** A patient who is having routine dental work done lies in the chair with arms crossed on his or her chest. (Do not *assume* that this means defensiveness.)
  I A possible interpretation is that the patient is trying to get comfortable.
  T Confirm your hypothesis by looking for other signs or by asking, "How do you feel, Mr. Baker?"
- **S** The dentist's gaze wanders as the hygienist is explaining why some changes in the tray set-up are desirable. (Do not assume that the dentist does not care.)
  I It might be reasonable to expect that the dentist is thinking of something else.
  T Test this interpretation, "I'd like to hear your thoughts, Dr. Green."

Eye Contact

Table 6–5 summarizes the important and varied roles that eye contact plays in communication.[3] Gaze functions primarily to provide context and amplify the meaning of spoken language and can perform all functions of verbal comunication, with the exception of transmitting information. In interpersonal communication, the average length of eye contact is only about three seconds, with speakers maintaining contact about twice as long as listeners.

TABLE 6–5. FUNCTIONS OF EYE CONTACT

Function	Applications
Regulates verbal communication	Indicates willingness to communicate; at end of sentence invites response; if strong and prolonged, demands response
Reflects topic interest	Pleasant topics involve more eye contact and little or none for embarrassing and sensitive topics; persuasive communication increases gaze
Mediates rapport	Increased eye contact is associated with warmth and friendliness; longer gazing is appropriate when listener is searching for feedback or speaking with a stigmatized individual, i.e., handicapped
Expresses emotion	Exaggerated gaze (staring) shows hostility; fear can be read in the eyes but not anger, disgust, or other emotions
Reflects status	Modest gaze at persons of very high status is appropriate; maximum gaze at higher status individuals; minimum gaze at lower status persons
Compensates for proximity	Eye contact increases with distance
Reflects personal characteristics	Extroverts display more eye contact; women gaze more at others but are quicker to avoid mutual eye contact

The Face

The fact that the upper face is visible throughout dental treatment makes it a potentially valuable source of information. In the give and take of conversation, facial expressions regulate conversation, such as slightly opening one's mouth to signal a desire to speak; "flirting" to get attention; or expressing surprise, doubt, or puzzlement to direct others to clarify their thoughts without actually interrupting.

The major use of facial expressions appears to be in conveying emotions. Multiple expressions can be conveyed simultaneously and recognizable changes can occur as fast as twice per second.[3] Emotions such as fear and sadness are most reliably registered in the eyes, the brows, and the forehead. Disgust and anger reside in the mouth and cheeks, whereas surprise and happiness are expressed over the entire face. This localization of facial expression of emotions is important in dental treatment. With instruments or rubber dams obscuring vision of the lower third of the face, clues to disgust and anger are likely to be missed.

The Body

In general, people are less sensitive to changes in their body than in their face, and they exercise less conscious control for masking or distortion. Muscle tone and posture are useful sources of information available to dental professionals. Some signs that are often taken to represent low self-esteem in patients include picking at oneself, scratching, cleaning nails, and twirling hair. Crossed arms and legs have become popularly identified with defensiveness. But this is only part of a complex of nonverbal behaviors that must be monitored for consistency. Facing the speaker, smiling, nodding, maintaining a relaxed facial expression or one that accurately and appropriately responds to the speaker, all reflect a lack of defensiveness. Exaggerated responsiveness with large and frequent gestures are a sign of needed approval.[2]

ACTING PROFESSIONALLY

Because nonverbal communication is so rich, subtle, and spontaneous, the only way to act consistently like a professional is to be one. The blend of confidence, caring, and warmth that is expected of professionals can be heightened or even faked, but only for short periods of time and at a cost in terms of energy. The following suggestions for enhancing the image of professionals should be practiced with a friend or in front of a mirror. Communication that is not genuine can be detected and is quite damaging to rapport.

The components recognized by most people as indicative of warmth include moving or leaning forward, eye contact, smiling, and facilitative behavior such as head nodding or saying "um hum." To strengthen the perceptions of confidence and trustworthiness, use a relaxed posture, expansive movements, reserve in showing facial emotion, pauses prior to speaking, and speech with good voice modulation and reasonable volume. In general, both respect and professionalism can be communicated by sensitivity to and application of give and take while talking and by appropriate responses to patients' communication. Certainly, interrupting patients or failing to react to their nonverbal expressions of strong emotions will erode rapport.

One behavior that does not express professionalism is the practice of arriving quickly and breathlessly to greet a patient. This may communicate that the operator is important and busy. Unfortunately, it also expresses that the patient is not important and that the professional is not in control.

TOUCHING

Touch is an integral part of dental care. Positioning the patient's head, assistance in and out of the chair, and chance contact at the front desk are some examples. As Table 6–6 illustrates, there are five categories of touching, and each has its own set of rules. When the rules, which may not be consciously known by patients or professionals, are broken, it is awkward and rapport may suffer.

Professional Touching

The contact with patients and co-workers that is an inescapable part of rendering care is called professional touching. Retracting cheeks, positioning radiographic film, and registering bites are examples. The contact is stereotyped and predictable, the professional devotes full attention to the task, introductory or explanatory remarks are often made, and eye contact is avoided.

TABLE 6–6. TYPES OF TOUCHING BEHAVIOR

Type	Circumstances	Behavior
Professional	In context of performing service, assisting patient into chair	Stereotyped, formal, explained, eye contact and social conversation limited
Accidental	In close quarters, unintentional bumps, narrow hallways, while working	Rigid body and posture, excuse offered, avoid social gestures
Social	In giving advice, information, trying to persuade; postoperative instructions; at patient dismissal	Toucher is usually of higher status and wants to influence other's behavior; confined to "insensitive" areas such as arm, shoulders, and back
Emotional	"Unmasks" signals that normal verbal and status roles are temporarily suspended; patient is choked with emotion	Willingness to listen and accept uncritically full emotional message
Therapeutic	Every aspect of health care delivery, but particularly at chairside	Warmth, gentleness, congruity of verbal and nonverbal aspects of communication

Accidental Touching

When people are crowded into an elevator or at a party, when miscalculations result in inadvertent bumps, or when two people reach for the same thing at the same time, the result is accidental touching. The rules appropriate for such situations are a brief apology, efforts to avoid further contact, and often an exaggerated rigid posture. Although eye contact is established it should not be prolonged.

Social Touching

Social touching is stereotypical contact designed to reduce "psychological" distance. The handshake shows trust and mutual respect. This type of touching usually accompanies giving advice or information, asking a favor, or trying to "get closer" in some other way. In a dental office it happens while greeting patients, when advising patients on homecare or postoperative instructions, or immediately after soliciting cooperation in situations where the dental professional wants something.

Social touching follows the conventions of social status.[8] Women are touched more than men and children are touched most frequently. The backs of hands and arms, shoulders, and the back are places where social touching is most likely to occur and least likely to be misunderstood. Touching the top of the head or the bottom communicates extreme status, as does a patting motion.

Emotional Touching

On occasion patients or co-workers are so choked with emotions such as grief, despair, or frustration that normal communication is impossible. Emotional touching is used by some professionals under these circumstances to signal that the customary status and social rules may be suspended momentarily.[9] Emotional touching includes hugging, taking another's hands in yours, and quickly grabbing another's arm, and it carries with it an obligation to listen empathetically and supportively to any emotional outpouring.

Therapeutic Touching

Physical contact with patients may be part of the cure itself. This might be defined liberally as the care shown in adjusting the head rest or the positive attitude developed through gentle instrumentation. Most faith healing involves the "laying on of hands." There are numerous studies stressing the curative aspects of communication, particularly touch, in the nursing field.[10–12]

CASE: THE STAND UP STAFF MEETING

The morning staff meeting to review cases in Dr. Warren's office was in progress. The dentist was standing in the lab facing the supply cabinets with a stack of records on the counter in front of him and his back to the rest of the staff. Paula Barker, the chairside assistant, was making a cup of instant coffee. The part-time assistant, Joanne Chang, sat on a stool watching the dentist's back in a rather distracted manner. After looking at several radiographs, Dr. Warren, without turning around, said in a complaining tone, "Where is the day sheet?" He abruptly walked out of the room without waiting for an answer. He returned a moment later, and looking around, he announced to no one in particular, "I known I've seen it somewhere." He rummaged in the charts again then slapped his forehead, "See, I told you I'd seen it."

The dentist asked several questions of the chairside assistant, still without facing anyone. Each time, the assistant began her answer tentatively, "Well, you know, Dr. Warren, . . ." He accepted each piece of information with a grunt, "ummmm . . .," or an exaggerated drop of the chart on the pile.

Martha Cunningham, the receptionist, entered and hung up her coat. No one greeted her. Finally, Dr. Warren turned around and leaned back against the counter with his arms crossed and a chart in one hand. He announced in a very loud voice, "Now that we're all finally here, there's something I want to say. I've got a chart here," as he waved it broadly, "with no write up and no billing information. This sort of thing is happening all the time and I'm not very happy."

He dropped the chart on the counter but continued to scowl at the receptionist who was busy making some coffee. "But, Dr. Warren," interjected the chairside assistant, "Martha couldn't have filed that chart. That's the one that's been missing for a week. We looked for it all yesterday. I don't know how you got it . . ."

As Paula Baker was speaking, the dentist was nodding in exaggerated agreement with a fed-up look on his face. Finally, he raised his hand to interrupt her, saying, "I know. I know. But what I'm talking about is the need for a general system." He handed the chart to the receptionist.

She took it and looked through it for a minute or two, straightening the inserts and centering the paper clip that was holding a note on top. Finally, without looking up she replied in a very emotionless voice, "It won't work."

She looked up abruptly as Dr. Warren frowned and almost spat back, "And why not?" She looked down at the chart again, took out a radiograph and reinserted it so that the label was clear, and answered softly, "It's just too complicated."

Paula Baker had been leaning forward at each pause and now she began, "Well, Dr. Warren, . . ." but the dentist spoke quickly and loudly and asked the part-time assistant, "I don't believe it. What do you think, Joanne?" The auxiliary opened her eyes and mouth suddenly and bolted upright, then slumped and shrugged her shoulders with a "palms out" gesture of her hands.

Paula Baker ventured once more, "Well . . ." But the dentist cut her off by taking the chart from the receptionist and handing it to the assistant with instructions to "do something about this."

ANALYSIS

The dentist in this case used nonverbal communication to control the flow of information and the status within the group. He avoided eye contact, a principle means of signaling that channels are open for communication, until he had something he felt was important to say. Then his direct and loud paralanguage demanded a response. His nonverbals controlled when others were permitted to talk, and he was effective in interrupting others, pretending agreement and using conspicuous hand gestures.

Martha Cunningham expressed a double message when she answered that a chart monitoring system would be too complex. Her tentative tone and lack of eye contact were not consistent with her firm verbal reply. Perhaps she feared retaliation but most likely she knows, as does the assistant, that the dentist will sabotage any system. The receptionist's constant straightening of things in the chart, in this case, was a habit that was not intended to communicate any information.

Several gestures substituted for spoken messages. The dentist slapping his forehead is one example, although perhaps overdone as he realizes he has been criticizing others for his own mistake of misplacing the day sheet. Joanne Chang's shrug and hand gestures express both uncertainty and a "why me?" attitude. The fact that she chose a nonverbal response is consistent with a posture of noninvolvement.

REFERENCES

1. Mehrabian, A. *Silent messages*. Belmont, Calif.: Wadsworth, 1971.
2. Knapp, M.L. *Nonverbal communication in human interaction* (2nd ed.). New York: Holt, Rinehart and Winston, 1978.
3. Ekman, P., & Friesen, W.V. *Unmasking the face: A guide to recognizing emotions from facial clues*. Englewood Cliffs, New Jersey: Prentice Hall, 1975.

4. Johnson, H.G., Ekman, P., & Friesen, W.V. Communicative body movements; American emblems. *Semiotica*, 1975, 15, 335–353.
5. Wiemann, J.M., & Knapp, M.L. Turn-taking in conversation. *Journal of Communication*, 1975, 25, 75–92.
6. Hall, E.T. *The hidden dimension.* Garden City, New Jersey: Doubleday, 1969.
7. Meisels, M., & Dosey, M. Personal space, anger, arousal and psychological defense. *Journal of Personality*, 1971, 39, 333–334.
8. Henley, N.M. *Body politics: Power sex, and nonverbal communication.* Englewood Cliffs, New Jersey: Prentice Hall, 1977.
9. Goffman, E. *The presentation of self in everyday life.* Garden City, New York: Doubleday, 1959.
10. Borelli, M.D., & Heidt, P. (Eds.). *Therapeutic touch.* New York: Springer, 1981.
11. Hammond, D.C., Hepworth, D.H., & Smith, V.G. *Improving therapeutic communication: A guide for developing effective techniques.* San Francisco: Jossey-Bass, 1979.
12. Lore, A. *Effective therapeutic communication.* Bowie, Md: Robert J. Brady, 1981.

EXERCISES

6–1. Watch television for a while with the sound off. Judge how confident you are about what you think the speakers (a) are saying, (b) how they feel, (c) how they relate to each other, liking and status, and (d) what kind of people they are, trusting, sophisticated, confident, and so on. Which of these characteristics are easy to judge from nonverbals and which are hard?

6–2. In a typical interpersonal interaction, such as a patient visit or lunch with a friend, take a systematic inventory of nonverbal cues. First focus on the eyes and eye contact. Next observe the entire face, then the speaker's posture and gestures, followed by the vocal messages, and lastly the context or general circumstances. Are the messages consistent? Which are the most believable and easily read components of communication? Now test your interpretation by paraphrasing what you see and hear and ask whether it is accurate.

6–3. Working with your learning partner, repeat the exercise above and find out what information and impressions you are communicating without being aware of them.

6–4. Compare the paralanguage, facial expressions, and gestures of local and national news commentators. Which gives you the greater sense of confidence and why?

6–5. Work with your learning partner or with someone who observes your interactions with others on a daily basis. For one week, each of you should prepare a list of nonverbal characteristics that express professionalism and a list of nonverbals that undermine the professional image. Discuss the lists and agree upon the changes you would like to make. Arrange for a nonverbal cue such as a thumbs up gesture or a "gun to the head" motion to signal "good" or "bad." Whenever you or your partner observe one of the behaviors targeted for improvement, the appropriate emblem should be given.

6–6. Practice reflecting. Select a time such as one evening when you regularly interact with a spouse, children, or roommate. "Listen" simultaneously on the verbal and the nonverbal channels until a double-level message is received. Reflect back your confusion over the inconsistency without stating or implying that you are blaming or condemning.

6–7. See if you can use social touching as an effective substitute for verbal communication. You might be able to show another person that you are interested in what they are saying, that you are supportive or sympathetic, or that you want some attention. Now repeat the same kind of message, with another person, but accompany your social touching with appropriate words.

DISCUSSION OF EXERCISES

6–1. Most people find it difficult, if not impossible, to do more than guess at the information component of communication based only on nonverbals. Personality and status are often evident in posture, timing, and closeness of the speakers. Emotions are the component of communication easiest to judge from nonverbals. The face and posture are good clues.

6–2. Some people find that they seldom are aware of anything beyond the verbal message. Others find that they are skilled at and tend to focus on eyes, face, or the body. Being able to identify components of messages is *not* the same as being able to use them. Typically those individuals most skilled in using nonverbal patterns to improve communication are unconscious of their own behavior and may not be able to "intellectualize" it.

6–3. Compare what your partner picks up with what you are aware of communicating. Repeat the exercise and see to what extent you can become conscious of your nonverbals. You may find that as you focus on one channel of communication another, such as uneven speech, betrays your efforts.

6–4. Most people find the measured, firm, and confident speech of national news reports more professional than local ones. There is also a built-in formality because of their working alone as opposed to being part of a team.

6–5. This is an example of using nonverbals to control verbal communication. It happens frequently in normal conversation. It is important in the exercise not to let patients or others see the signals or become distracted.

6–6. A good reflecting expression conveys both the verbal message and the inconsistent nonverbal message. True experts can sometimes reflect by repeating the verbal message with a surprised or puzzled look, although caution is needed to avoid sarcasm.

6–7. Social touching that is consistent with an appropriate verbal message is an effective illustrator, provided that the proper rules are observed. Professional and accidental touching cannot take the place of words—it requires certain verbal expressions to place it in context.

7

Persuasion and Motivation

There are numerous situations in which persuasion and motivation can make dental practice more effective and enjoyable. Patients who value oral health and learn to take an active role in it will also elect better care, make more referrals, and be a pleasure in the office. By contrast, some patients must be convinced to remain quiet during treatment, arrive for appointments on time, pay for treatment, and follow minimal postsurgical procedures. There are also times when persuasive and motivational communication is needed to adjust staff hours, office policies, and coworkers' attitudes.

This chapter describes how persuasion works and illustrates ten basic rules for effective persuasion. The chapter concludes with a discussion of the resources and limits of persuasion available to dental professionals.

Persuasion means using communication to change attitudes or move others to action. Sometimes the term motivation is used when describing a short-term behavior change brought about by persuasive communication. Persuasive communication considers the integrity of others and is aimed at behavior and its positive attitudes. Those who are persuaded or motivated understand and appreciate desired action and will not feel "used." Power, on the other hand, disregards beliefs and seeks only changed behavior.

HOW PERSUASION WORKS

Let us assume the dentist wants to convince the new assistant of the value of working staggered lunch hours. There are four general approaches available in this situation.

- Appeal to rapport: "I'm asking you as a friend, or an employer."
- Appeal to consequences: "This will give you more flexibility."
- Appeal to values: "We need to work out something that is fair to everybody."
- Appeal to consistent behavior and attitudes: "You will take the early shift for the first week and we'll see how it works out."

The four approaches shown in Table 7–1 are based on the fact that people want to be consistent. We angle to hold attitudes or adopt behaviors that are compatible with our friends and those in

TABLE 7–1. FOUR APPROACHES TO PERSUASION BASED ON NEED FOR CONSISTENCY

Approach	Need	Example
Appeal to rapport	Agree with friends and those in authority	"You could do me a favor." "Would you listen to a little advice from someone who's been there?"
Appeal to consequences	Make choices that lead to desired results	"That approach has been known to backfire." "If you look at it as an investment it wouldn't seem so hard."
Appeal to values	Preserve fundamental or cherished beliefs	"I know you want to do what's right for your child." "I thought you said that efficiency was the key."
Appeal to consistent behavior and attitudes	Allow attitudes to become consistent with behavior *and* behavior to become consistent with attitudes	"Now that you've stopped smoking don't you feel better?" "If you want to feel better you can stop smoking."

positions of authority, that lead to desirable results, that agree with our fundamental values, and that keep our behavior and attitudes consistent with each other.[1] This view has the singular advantage over other theories of persuasion of guaranteeing that the integrity of patients and co-workers will not be violated and hence that persuasion is built on a firm foundation.[2]

Appeal to Rapport

Cooperative behavior and pro-health attitudes in the dental office are often built on interpersonal relations. The need to belong and to socialize is a powerful motivator,[3] and an alert professional can use this to advantage. Most patients keep appointments and pay bills simply because they are asked to and because they value their relationship with the dentist and the staff. Rapport, the mutual extending of trust and suspension of judgment, is part of the foundation for persuasion and motivation. Respected friends are more persuasive than strangers—even very logical and articulate ones.

Appeal to Consequences

None of us has thought through all the consequences of everything we think we want. Patients certainly cannot be expected to know the complete effects of dental care or neglect. Persuasion is often a matter of pointing out the hidden negative results or the unknown benefits in the available options. Dental professionals are uniquely qualified to perform this service of helping patients "think through" dental care.

- *(Dentist to patient)* "Please don't make any sudden moves for the next two minutes while this impression is hardening. Movement might cause distortion and that would result in a denture that fits badly."
- *(Receptionist to dentist)* "I think we had better set a regular time for taking emergencies. The last week has been a real mess."
- *(Dentist to spouse)* "You shouldn't be so down on Dorothy. Patients tell me she's the best hygienist I've had in years."

Appeal to Values

"Attitudes" and "values" are not synonymous terms.[2] Attitudes are limited and temporary feelings toward individual, relatively unimportant things such as cars, television personalities, or even dental care. Values, such as fairness, morality, industry, authority, and respect for others, become part of our identity and are changed slowly and with great difficulty.

When attitudes or behaviors are inconsistent with fundamental values we feel discomfort, embarrassment, or anxiety, and this uneasiness can be a powerful motivating force.[1] Pointing out discrepancies, without being judgmental, is persuasive because others will modify what they are doing or how they feel about things to preserve consistency with their values.

- *(Dentist to colleague)* "How can you support Wilbur for the State Board. You know how he feels about manpower and the denturists." (Assumes a strong value of professional identification)
- *(Assistant to colleague)* "But you have to ask for a raise. You had to borrow to make last month's rent." (Assumes strong need to earn a living)
- *(Hygienist to patient)* "Because you want to keep these teeth I'm going to demonstrate an effective means you can use to clean them." (Assumes strong dental health value)

Appeal to Consistent Behavior and Attitudes

Most people feel awkward when it is pointed out that their attitudes and behavior are inconsistent. When dental professionals eat candy they joke about plaque or their diet. Smokers avoid discussing lung cancer. Although it is commonly assumed that behavior can be modified by first shifting attitudes, the opposite approach is just as likely to be effective. Generally, it is the weaker of attitudes or behavior that will be changed to return to consistency. It is both possible and practical to change behavior first in the confident expectation that consistent attitudes will follow. For example, once patients have selected a treatment plan, they tend to develop or pick up attitudes that justify their choice. Everything done in an effective dental practice need not be justified in advance.

TEN RULES OF PERSUASION

In addition to the four general approaches to persuasion just presented, there are ten specific rules that can be applied.[4–6] Using these rules by themselves will not guarantee results, but they do increase the chances of predictable outcomes (Table 7–2).

TABLE 7–2. TEN RULES OF PERSUASION

Rule	Consequences of Breaking the Rule
1. Accept others' views	Listeners' emotions will become a barrier to communication Speaker appears to be closed-minded and untrustworthy
2. Reduce resistance	Listener becomes more stressed Reduced communication Listener becomes defensive
3. Be honest	Messages sound ungenuine, unconvincing Discovered deception creates resentment and erodes future confidence
4. Avoid scare tactics	Listeners reduce threat through undesirable means such as fantasy and avoidance
5. Do not oversell	Negative attitudes will develop Suspicion may develop
6. Do not undersell	Compliance will not be achieved Listener will be more defensive and harder to persuade next time
7. Do not undercharge	Listener will place a low value on services that are easily obtained
8. The power of silence	Listener has no opportunity to make a choice Suspicion arises from overselling
9. Post-decision persuasion	Listener remains uncomfortable Chance of reversing decision or poor follow-through exists
10. Decisionmaker's responsibility	Listener feels less committed to decisions Speaker may be liable if recommended action fails

1. Accept Others' Views

Empathy is valuable in the early stages of persuasion because it shows openness and builds rapport. At the same time, it helps control potentially obstructive emotions and reveals others' values. Acknowledging contrary opinions assures that the subject has been fully considered and demonstrates an open mind. Mentioning without judgment that alternative views exist prevents their being used by others at a later, critical point in the discussion. It becomes increasingly important to listen empathically when dealing with informed persons and with complex issues.[7]

- *(Dentist to assistant seeking a raise)* "I do understand that some of the dentists in town are paying more."
- *(Assistant to dentist reluctant to give a raise)* "I know you're concerned about how long I've been here."

2. Reduce Resistance

Everyone wants dental health and quality treatment. Patients are held back by fear of pain, inconvenience, cost, uncertainty, and many other personal factors. There are thus two strategies for dental professionals to promote health behavior: Emphasize the advantages of dental health or reduce the disadvantages that are impeding it.

Reducing obstacles to healthy behavior is generally the preferred technique. Explore and dissipate patients' fear and uncertainty. Educate patients about convenience and cost-saving opportunities. As resistance crumbles, the positive attitudes that have always been there will manifest themselves in desired behavior. Patients have been so bombarded with health messages that resistance-reducing messages offer a wiser tact. The professional thus assumes a helping role and can create a more relaxed and receptive atmosphere.

- *(Receptionist to patient)* "We will allow you to make the payment in three equal parts."
- *(Hygienist to patient)* "Let me show you how you can cut flossing time by half."

3. Be Honest

Lying or misleading patients and co-workers may achieve short-term compliance, but the overall effect is apt to be negative. When there is an inconsistency between a persuasive message and non-verbal facial expressions, gestures, and intonation, the message is not believable. The listener is confused and the speaker is no longer seen as genuine.[8] When a misleading message is believed and the deception is later discovered, trust is eroded and future messages are suspect. It is necessary to mention all sides of an argument if it is likely that others will hear them eventually.

4. Avoid Scare Tactics

Scare tactics do provoke changes in behavior and attitudes, but the changes are not always the ones desired. Patients who are frightened and co-workers who are threatened can be expected to seek comfort in the most convenient way possible, though not necessarily the most constructive way.[9] For example, if office members are told that their performance "had better improve if they wish to keep their jobs," they can mentally excuse themselves for just having a bad day or can forget that they heard the message. The ultimate escape from anxiety-provoking messages is avoidance.

Staff members avoid each other's company. Patients find other dentists.

When scare tactics must be used, the following precautions should be exercised: (1) scare tactics are the motivational tool of last resort; (2) the amount of anxiety created should be kept to the minimum necessary; and (3) an acceptable means of reducing stress should be offered immediately.[10]

- *(Dentist to patient)* "The tests are not as good as I had hoped for, but I have some things that we can do that should help."
- *(Dentist to hygienist)* "We can't go on like this. You are consistently taking too long with the prophies. Let's see if we can't figure this out."
- *(Dentist to adolescent patient)* "Now if you don't wear this headgear every day, it won't help you. Let's have another trial run."

5. Do Not Oversell

Excessive persuasive pressure is called coercion and although it achieves compliant behavior, it also has negative side effects. Overselling results in unfavorable attitudes and erodes trust.

Making a patient "an offer he can't refuse" will secure temporary cooperation, but it will not be enthusiastic cooperation. Which patient will have the most positive attitude toward the practice: the one who pays the bill because the receptionist mentions the cost of materials used or the one contacted by a collection agency? Overselling also invites suspicion. A patient who is ready for the recommended therapy can be scared off by an unnecessarily aggressive sales pitch.

6. Do Not Undersell

Underselling is actually worse than overselling. The desired behavior is not achieved and negative attitudes are also generated. A common mistake in persuasion is to assume that there is "no harm in trying." An example is underselling the use of floss as part of effective oral hygiene. When this happens, the patient's defenses and excuses are activated with no change in behavior. Subsequent attempts to persuade this patient must deal with the additional resistance the patient created to defend against the ineffective presentation.

When resistance is encountered, the best strategy is to assess whether it is likely that the listener will ever cooperate. If not, persuasion should be discontinued. If the determination cannot be made with confidence, the persuader should proceed slowly until it can be judged whether and how cooperation might be won.

7. Do Not Undercharge

If there is no obvious external reason for behavior, then an internal value exists. If patients willingly pay more for care, they will develop more positive attitudes in order to remain consistent with their behavior. If dentists charge little or nothing for homecare instruction, patients will judge it to be of diminished value.

Patients, on the other hand, cannot be made to appreciate dentistry simply by raising fees. Internal values adjust to compensate for behavior only when the behavior is voluntary.[1]

8. The Power of Silence

The conclusion of most persuasive communication is a clear period of silence. Patients cannot agree with a dental professional who is too busy talking to let the patient answer. The opportunity to respond to persuasion should be clear enough for the listener to recognize that a response is expected. This will make the listener more committed to the response. Following this pattern also protects against the danger of talking too long, overselling, and arousing suspicion and defensiveness.

- *(Hygienist to patient)* "Based on what I've told you, you will have to tell me what you prefer. (pause)"
- *(Dentist to patient)* "I have summarized the advantages and disadvantages, but the decision is yours. (pause)"

9. Post-Decision Persuasion

Perhaps the most important time to make a persuasive comment is just after the listener has reached a decision. Patients and coworkers need reassurance that the actions they have chosen are correct.

When it is difficult to reach a conclusion, tension builds. A patient who wavers between an amalgam restoration and an inlay must recognize merits and drawbacks in each option. Deciding on the inlay does not reduce the advantages of the amalgam restoration. Dental professionals can help to relieve this uneasiness by focusing on the benefits of the chosen action or the problems with the choices not selected. Reducing this discomfort will put the listener at ease and reduce the risk of flip-flop decisions or ones that are only followed in a half-hearted fashion.

- *(Dentist to patient)* "Yes, I think that is a sound choice in your situation."
- *(One assistant to another)* "I'm glad you're going back to school. The way you described it, it really sounds like that's what you want to do."

10. Decision Maker's Responsibility
Patients cannot transfer responsibility for decisions affecting their health, but some trap dental professionals into making decisions for them. "I don't know. You just tell me what to do, Doctor," is so tempting for professionals who seek control over interpersonal relations or who think they see a chance to save a few seconds time. This response, however, may lead to legal complications when the recommended therapy fails. Moreover, when not actively involved in the decision, patients tend to assume less responsibility.

When patients attempt to transfer responsibility they should be politely reminded that it is the patients' right and obligation to decide about their own health. "I will be happy to give you all the information I can. But you know that this must ultimately be your decision." Direct recommendations should be avoided. One procedure that helps dental professionals to avoid making unwarranted recommendations is to phrase responses to include an "if" clause.

- *(Dentist to patient) "If* that tooth is left untreated, it will probably abscess and cause you a great deal of pain."
- *(Hygienist to patient) "If* my son had that type of overbite, I would probably seek more advice."

USES OF PERSUASION

It is ethical to influence patients' and co-workers' attitudes and motivate them to modify their behavior. In fact, it is impossible not to influence others, either by example or by refusing to comment. The real issue is the means used to influence others. All of the techniques presented in this chapter are consistent with maintaining the integrity of both dental staff and patients. Other methods for changing attitudes and behavior fail in all but the expedient present. As expressed by Gerard Nierenberg,[5] "People do not resist change; they resist being changed."

Available Resources

Dentists and the office staff have certain special resources for influencing patient attitudes. These strengths include expertise and authority, rapport and trust, and teamwork (Table 7–3).

Limits of Persuasion

It is confusing and often frustrating that dental professionals have so much influence over the behavior and attitudes of patients in the dental office and so little influence when patients leave. Later chapters present methods for modifying behavior outside the dental office. It must be remembered that persuasion and motivation are means of achieving only short-term changes. Whether such modifications eventually develop into substantial values and habits depends on whether they serve patients' fundamental needs by proving meaningful and helpful.

The most powerful resource for persuasion available to dental professionals is their expertise, particularly with regard to patient behavior. This resource, however, is limited because influence is focused on dental behavior. In other aspects of patients' lives dental professionals have little influence. When dental needs come in conflict with other patient needs, there is little the dentist or staff can do. This is one reason why diet and homecare are so difficult to modify.

CASE: PROPER EXPOSURE OF A PATIENT TO DIAGNOSTIC RADIOGRAPHS

The assistant, Valery Martins, said, "Alright, Mrs. Stattlemeyer, we are going to take some x-rays so that Dr. Maynard can check for cavities between the teeth."

TABLE 7–3. PERSUASIVE RESOURCES IN THE DENTAL OFFICE

Resource	Foundation	Precaution
Expertise and authority	Dental professionals know what is happening in patients' mouths; patients are uncertain	Avoid justification or discussion of your qualification
Rapport and trust	Dentists enjoy high level of general trust; there is less need for justifications and explanations; "credit" is extended by patients	Avoid suspicion that recommendation is motivated by income or convenience; avoid undermining patient trust in co-workers
Teamwork	An office staff with same messages, philosophy, and approach to patients enhances trust and relaxes patients	Inconsistencies have opposite and damaging effects

As she approached the patient, apron in hand, she noticed a scowl on Mrs. Stattlemeyer's face. "You look concerned," she suggested.

"Well, I don't really know. But I've heard all this stuff on the television about microwave radiation, and congenital defects, and all that . . ."

Valery put down the apron and drew up a stool to sit facing Mrs. Stattlemeyer. "You sound worried about ill-effects of excess radiation."

"Well, shouldn't I be? I mean, isn't it true what they say about it causing cancer and birth defects?"

"Yes, Dr. Maynard has had several staff meetings to talk about this. We've read some of the literature and we've had the machines tested. We have been very concerned about this ourselves, and it's right for you to be concerned, too. Dr. Maynard told us he only recommends x-rays when it is important for a thorough examination and diagnosis."

"Well," asked Mrs. Stattelmeyer, "what are the chances of anything bad happening?"

"Under normal circumstances the odds of any negative effects are so small that we say there is no practical risk. Now if you are pregnant or if you have just had some x-rays then we would have to consider the situation."

"At my age it's not very likely that I would be pregnant, is it? And I haven't been to a dentist in eight years." The patient sighed and looked inquiringly at Valery Martins.

"You still seem hesitant, Mrs. Stattlemeyer."

"Oh, I don't know. It sounds okay. But, well, you know my neighbor down the street just died of cancer. There's so much of it going around."

"You're worried about the x-rays causing cancer . . ."

"Well, you didn't say anything about that, and it seems to me I read something about it."

"Yes there have been several studies and the results have been unclear. But one thing we know is that there is no evidence that the kind of equipment we use here can cause cancer. I promise you, Mrs. Stattlemeyer, I am very concerned myself because I use this equipment many times every day. If I had any doubts then I wouldn't be doing this.

"But the decision is really yours. Based on what I have told you about the safety of the equipment and the advantage it provides Dr. Maynard for diagnosing your case, you will have to tell me what you prefer."

There was a moment's hesitation then the patient said, "Oh, sure, go ahead."

Valery dropped the apron over Mrs. Stattlemeyer and began to position the cone. "You know I was as concerned as you were about the safety of x-rays. But when Dr. Maynard explained what the studies mean and when I remembered that this equipment and the procedures we use are approved and regularly checked by the state, I stopped worrying. How do you feel about your decision now?"

"Yeah, you're right. It's so confusing these days. But I trust your judgment."

ANALYSIS

In this example, Valery Martins used each of the four approaches to persuasion in order to motivate Mrs. Stattlemeyer. She built *rapport* through empathic responses and relating her own concerns. This rapport was used as personal influence—"if I had any doubts then I wouldn't be doing this." The assistant also appealed to *consequences*—"Dr. Maynard can check for cavities between the teeth." The appeal to *values* was based on the impression that Mrs. Stattlemeyer places faith in authority. Valery Martins referred to the authority of the dentist, of scientific studies, and state regulations. The foundation of the assistant's motivational strategy was to convince the patient to permit the radiographs. She did not attempt to change the patient's attitudes about the effects of radiation in general. The assistant knows that once the patient agrees to radiographs, her *attitude will shift in the direction of her behavior.*

REFERENCES

1. Festinger, L. *A theory of cognitive dissonance.* Stanford, Calif.: Stanford University Press, 1957.
2. Brown, R. *Social psychology.* New York: The Free Press, 1965.
3. Maslow, A.H. *Motivation and personality.* New York: Harper, 1954.
4. Bradley, B.E. *Fundamentals of speech communication: The credibility of ideas* (3rd ed.). Dubuque, Iowa: William C. Brown, 1974.
5. Nierenberg, G.I. *How to give and receive advice.* New York: Pocket Books, 1975.
6. Verderber, R.F. *Communicate* (2nd. ed.). Belmont, Calif.: Wadsworth, 1978.
7. Brown, R. *Words and things: An introduction to language.* New York: The Free Press, 1958.
8. Satir, V. *Peoplemaking.* Palo Alto, Calif.: Science and Behavior Books, 1972.
9. Lazarus, R.S. *Psychological stress and the coping process.* New York: McGraw-Hill, 1966.
10. Pervin, L.A. The need to predict and control under conditions of threat. *Journal of Personality,* 1963, 31, 570–578.

EXERCISES

7–1. Think of the last argument you lost. Recall and write down who you were arguing with, what you wanted, how you went about it, and how you know that you lost the argument. Did you use any of the four basic appeals to rapport, consequences, values, or the consistency of behavior and attitudes? Did you use any of the ten basic rules?

7–2. Consider your answers to the first exercise and plot a general strategy for persuasion were you able to go back to the beginning of the argument.

7–3. Sometime during the coming week when you are in a persuasion situation, stop prior to beginning your message. Program yourself to ask at least three questions designed to diagnose the position from which the other person is coming. The questions will differ depending on the circumstances.

7–4. Plan four persuasive messages for the following hypothetical situation. You want the dentist to send you and another assistant to the University for a two-day continuing education course in nitrous oxide–oxygen analgesia. Write an appeal based on each of the four consistency approaches suggested in this chapter.

7–5. Read through the following brief case and identify instances where the ten rules of persuasion are violated.

Mr. Williams leaned forward blocking Patty's attempt to position the cone on the radiographic unit. "Hey, do I have a choice in this?"

In candid surprise Patty stopped and asked, "What do you mean? You don't want x-rays?"

Well, I'm not sure I do and I'm not sure I don't. I hear they can cause you to go sterile."

"Oh, come now, Mr. Williams," Patty said, putting her head on one side and stepping back. "Where did you hear that nonsense? This machine puts out no more radiation than you would get if you took an hour's sun bath in the mountains at Aspen. We need these x-rays to find interproximal caries and Dr. Parsons has a policy of not treating patients who refuse bitewings unless they sign a consent form waiving all legal rights to sue for problems that might arise. I really can't imagine though what the fuss is all about. Now put your head back, Mr. Williams. You can take my word for it, everything will be fine."

DISCUSSION OF EXERCISES

7–1. and 7–2. Most arguments are lost because they are failed attempts to control behavior through power rather than by locating a position in the person with whom one is arguing that can be used for one of the four consistency techniques. It is more natural for us to argue from what is rational or consistent for ourselves, but it is more effective to begin with what makes sense to our "opponent." Opponents are considered to be stubborn when they do not see the logic of our view and we are ineffective to the extent that we fail to see from where they are starting.

7–3. "How do you feel about . . ." and "I'm curious to know what you think . . ." are good general questions. Because the people with whom you are talking will eventually form a pattern of attitudes and behaviors that is consistent *from their point of view*, time can be saved and the likelihood of success increased by starting with an understanding of others' perspectives.

7–4. For example: (a) Appeal to rapport—"Sylvia and I need your help . . ." (b) Appeal to consequences—"This will make the office more effective . . ." (c) Appeal to values—"You have always said how every member of the staff is equally important . . ." (d) Appeal to consistent behavior and attitudes—"You'll be glad you let us do this."

7–5. The assistant failed to acknowledge Mr. Williams' concerns. In fact, she belittled them. She increased the patient's stress by offering counterarguments rather than weakening resistance to his concerns. Her use of technical language may have been misleading, and scare tactics contained a clear lie. In no jurisdiction in the United States can a patient waive his or her recourse to the law, no matter what they sign. Without even determining the nature and depth of Mr. Williams' concern, it is quite probable that Patty oversold her case. She might have succeeded in securing temporary compliance, but it is most likely that Mr. Williams will be suspicious, perhaps resentful of the way he is treated in this office. The assistant failed to allow the patient to make a decision. She assumed responsibility for the decision, "You can take my word for it."

Part II

TREATMENT ALLIANCE

In the dental office, communication is an investment. An initial expenditure of time and effort is made with an expectation that subsequent dental care will be faster, of better quality, and more pleasant. Communication is also the key to a successful treatment alliance. This alliance is the working relationship between patients and professionals and is fundamental to optimal dental care and oral health. It is based on realistic, mutual expectations and respected values. With effective communication, the patient will see that the professional cares and understands.

The next seven chapters discuss basic interpersonal communication skills in relation to the dental treatment alliance. Patient's emotional needs are discussed in "Anxiety, Anger, Depression, Apathy, and Impatience," then the unique intellectual and social backgrounds of "Children and Older Patients" are reviewed. The subsequent four chapters apply basic skills to specific dental situations in which communication plays a key role: "Interviewing and History Taking," "Treatment Plan and Informed Consent," "Compliance," which involves following recommendations, keeping appointments, and paying for services, and "Oral Hygiene Instruction." A final chapter in this section explores the impact of office design, environment, and printed matter on patient expectations and behavior.

The remainder of this introduction shows the benefits of sound treatment alliances and the need for customizing them.

SOUND TREATMENT ALLIANCES PAY OFF

Increased Job Satisfaction

Reports of stress and suicide among dentists and high turnover among auxiliaries contain a common theme—lack of satisfaction with the repetitive nature of technical tasks and, occasionally, frustration with patients.[1] Dentists often describe the toughest problems encountered as patients who make unreasonable demands, show a disappointing lack of regard for their own oral health, or stubbornly decline the quality of care that the dentist offers. Communication can be used to build better working relationships and reduce unrealistic expectations that are the source of so much stress.

Increased Busyness

Dental professionals can use communication skills to build busy practices of satisfied patients. When patients know what to expect and value what they receive, they are less reluctant to seek dental care. When patients feel their needs are not being met, they can become management problems. If the situation becomes bad enough, they may leave the practice. Techniques for diagnosing and responding to patients' needs enhance patient appreciation and may attract others who value effective relationships.

Fewer Lawsuits

The principle complaint in disciplinary actions and lawsuits against dentists revolves around fees and not the quality of technical care or accuracy of diagnosis.[2] Without a satisfactory treatment alliance, patients feel less obligated to implied contractual obligations. Late and incomplete payment, broken appointments, and disregard for professional advice are the result.

Patients Hold Key to Quality of Work

It is the patient who has final authority over the quality of therapy that the dentist is allowed to perform and over its maintenance. The recommended endodontic treatment and full crown coverage may be declined in favor of exodontia and a removable partial appliance by a patient who does not trust professionals or cannot be made to see the advantages of optimal care.

Time Savings

Paradoxically, communication can produce substantial time savings in a dental practice. Consider the typical time wasters: late arrivals, management problems, patients who must have instructions or explanations repeated, complaints, "redo's," and justifications. In these cases, as in dentistry in general, prevention is less costly than repair of neglect. Coming to an understanding about important expectations in advance requires some communication, but can save prolonged and often stressful encounters later.

Improved Patient Health

Communication can be directly therapeutic. In a hospital study involving operations such as appendectomies,[3] some patients were told what would be done and how they could be expected to feel during and following surgery, whereas others were left uninformed. Not only did the patients who had the benefit of a treatment alliance feel more positive toward the experience and the staff, they also required significantly less postsurgical analgesia and were discharged earlier.

CUSTOMIZED TREATMENT ALLIANCES

Reciprocal expectations and mutual values of patients and dental health professionals are vital to the treatment alliance. Some basic set of needs must be at least partially satisfied as a condition for continuing treatment.[4] When expectations are not met, communication becomes more difficult, unpredictable behavior increases, and patients leave the practice or dentists discharge their patients.

The expectations and values that constitute a treatment alliance are typically *assumed* rather than stated. Besides those noted in Table II–1, there are also cultural, personal, and situational variations.[5] Communication skills are needed for expressing expectations that professionals have for patient behavior ("You must control your gingival health before I can make the bridge"), learning what patients expect ("Doctor, would you please explain all the options again"), and making necessary adjustments ("I'm going to need more complete answers on this health history form in order to avoid problems later").

Every culture and subculture has its own standards for interpersonal relations. A young practitioner in a liberal suburb might dress casually and call patients by their first names. This would be

TABLE II–1. CORE EXPECTATIONS IN THE TREATMENT ALLIANCE

Expected of Dental Professionals	Expected of Patients
Eliminate pain Show courtesy and consideration Perform restorative procedures Offer informed consent Protect confidences and avoid embarrassing patient Keep costs and time within reasonable ranges	Give honest and complete answers to appropriate questions Be prompt Pay for services Follow through on recommended postoperative and homecare instructions

inappropriate in many other communities. In some socioeconomic groups, the standard of care, and therefore the kind of treatment expected by patients, may be less than ideal. Some dentists may not be able to deliver optimal care in such a neighborhood—too few patients would accept the terms of such an alliance.

There are also personal differences that affect treatment alliances. Some patients are unusually sensitive to pain; others are worried about cost. Some people are gregarious and suspicious of professionals who are reserved and formal. Uncomfortable feelings might also result when a retiring or business-like patient encounters a talkative office staff member.

Finally, there are situational factors that form an important part of the treatment alliance. A normally sociable patient may be ill, tired, or worried. To proceed in this case as though nothing has changed would risk irritating the patient. When the dentist is running late, patients are more likely to accept the tardy care if the dentist explains and asks permission.

Adult patients and professionals typically understand the core expectations of the treatment alliance and applicable cultural modifications. Personal and situational variations, however, require extra communication. Patients feel better when they are told how much time is required to perform a new procedure, what is to be done and how they can expect to feel, and the cost and how they are expected to pay. Unexpected complications and problems with office routine should not be kept from the patient. Some patients do announce that they are tired, in a hurry, afraid of being hurt, or concerned about cost. Many others hide these feelings or offer only subtle hints that the dental staff must interpret.

Sometimes, establishing a treatment alliance is made difficult by conflicting expectations. A patient may be going to the hygienist under the expectation that professional care is a complete substitute for personal responsibility. A patient may be seeking care only to eliminate acute pain and restore function at minimal cost, whereas the dentist may be accustomed to providing optimal care. Out of fear, a patient may be very brief and incomplete in answering questions about medical history or personal feelings. These cases require well-developed communication skills.

If significant differences between the expectations and the values of patients and dentists remain after a good-faith effort at communication, it is no failure to refer the patient to another practitioner.[6] The treatment alliance must preserve the dignity of both patients and professionals. An honest "agreement to disagree" is preferable to patients spreading unfavorable reports about their dentist. However, the communication skills presented in these chapters should help develop and maintain sound treatment alliances and ensure their benefits.

REFERENCES

1. Lange, A.L., Loupe, M.J., & Meskin, L.H. Professional satisfaction in dentistry. *Journal of the American Dental Association*, 1982, 104, 619–624.
2. de St. Georges, J.M. How to maximize your opportunities through third-party dentistry. *Practice Management*, 1982, 22, 16–21.
3. Egbert, L., Battit, G., Welch, C., & Bartlett, M. Reduction in postoperative pain by encouragement and instruction of patients. *New England Journal of Medicine*, 1964, 270, 825–827.
4. Enelow, A.J. & Swisher, S.N. *Interviewing and patient care.* New York: Oxford University Press, 1972.
5. Fredericks, M.A., Lobene, R.R., & Mundy, P. *Dental care in society: The sociology of dental health.* Jefferson, N.C.: McFarland, 1980.
6. American Dental Association. *ADA principles of ethics and code of professional conduct.* Chicago: American Dental Association, undated.

8

Anxiety, Anger, Depression, Apathy, and Impatience

Emotions are an inescapable aspect of dental care. Dental professionals are not psychiatrists, but they must be proficient in the rudimentary skills of recognizing their own and patients' moods and in discussing them to facilitate sound dental practice. The fundamental techniques presented in this chapter require surprisingly little time to use. Trying to ignore patients' feelings will not prevent disruptive emotions from compromising treatment or surfacing in conversations outside the office. It is not fair or productive for dentists and their staffs to be emotional doormats for their patients.

The strong emotions presented in this chapter all consititute natural defense systems.[1] Within bounds they are healthy protective reactions to threat of physical or psychological danger, including uncertainty, fatigue, lack of control, and status manipulation. The dental setting normally contains many such emotion-provoking situations. Typically, emotions in the dental office are appropriate and need not be curtailed. Failure to recognize legitimate feelings leads to dishonesty, fantasy, noncooperation, absenteeism, and rumor-mongering.[2] Similarly, inappropriate emotional reactions must be diagnosed, managed, and, when necessary, referred.

This chapter contains six sections. The five strong emotions—anxiety, anger, depression, apathy, and impatience—are defined and it is shown how each can be recognized. Dental factors likely to stimulate each emotion and consequences for communication are mentioned. Some do's and don't's are suggested for how these emotions can be managed. The sixth section deals specifically with the emotions of dental professionals. Their anger or impatience does not differ appreciably from that of patients but there are special conventions that apply to professionals displaying or discussing personal feelings.

ANXIETY

Detection

Anxious individuals look concerned, have difficulty sitting still, cannot concentrate, are easily distracted, breathe quickly and shallowly, may move their fingers or feet in repetitive patterns, and may perspire on the forehead or upper lip (Table 8–1). When talking, they are unsure of themselves and avoid making decisions or committing themselves to action. They talk too much and too rapidly with frequent changes of topic. They may also be very quiet, giving only minimal answers to direct questions and volunteering no information. Children may even fall asleep. There is also a tendency for anxious people to overreact. They might describe themselves as "nervous," "just a little on edge," or even "uncomfortable."[3]

Function

Anxiety is a signal that some threat to the person or self-image is present, and consequently the body's defenses are put on alert. Anxiety elicits several physiological reactions, i.e., accelerated

TABLE 8–1. CHARACTERISTICS OF ANXIETY

Function	Detection	Dental Sources
Signals danger and mobilizes defenses	Excessive random movement	Pain
	Rapid speech and respiration	Loss
	Overreaction	Disapproval
	Uncertainty	Uncertainty
	Tentativeness	Self-disclosure

Communication Problems	Management
Narrow attention	*Do:* Empathically understand, talk about it
Fixation on problems	*Don't:* Ignore, reassure
Regression to habits	

heart rate, dilated pupils, withdrawing blood from extremities and concentrating it internally, and release of hormones.[4] The resultant behavior is characteristic of people trying to protect themselves. It is also individually conditioned. Past experience plays a large role in determining what will be anxiety-provoking and how it will be expressed. Children are no more anxious than adults, but adults have merely learned ways of masking the more obvious signs of anxiety.

Dental Sources

There are obvious reasons for patients to be anxious in a dental office. Pain and unknown dangers are associated with probing, injecting, drilling, and cutting. Less obvious causes of dental anxiety involve cost, loss of function and appearance in extractions, disfiguration in periodontal and maxillofacial surgery, disapproval and ridicule from professionals for poor oral hygiene practices, discovery of the need for extensive work or of life-threatening conditions, disclosure of personal habits such as lip biting, and fear that patients will act inappropriately or be unable to control their own emotions.

Sometimes the mere lack of ground rules or established expectations causes anxiety. Some fears may be unfounded or based on misinformation, such as fear of being sexually assaulted. Some may be psychotic, as in identifying teeth with virility. Regardless of the source or rationale of patients' fears, the emotion of anxiety is absolutely real if present. If a dental professional says to a patient "You have nothing to be afraid of; stop worrying," it is the professional who is acting irrationally.

Patients often send confusing signals about their anxiety. For example, patients who are afraid that a long procedure means complications and discomfort might say that they are concerned about leaving on time to pick up the children. Often anxiety is disguised as aggression. "Is all of this really necessary?" or "Gracious, this is taking a long time" could be translated to "I'm worried about what you're doing." The most typical way of covering anxiety is to deny it and mask its symptoms. Patients who are trying especially hard to control their feelings become silent and rigid. Patients disguise their anxiety because they are uncertain how the professional will react to them.

Communication Problems

Anxiety is particularly disruptive in any aspect of dental care where gathering information or giving directions is involved. Anxiety focuses attention on the cause of concern and usually results in overdependence on habitual and well-learned behavior.[5] A patient who is fixated on possible oral cancer will give incomplete information on the health history, will not pay attention or may be uncooperative during the examination, and will not hear much of what is being said. Anxious patients are poor candidates for homecare instruction and they have difficulty remembering even the simplest of postsurgical instructions.

Management

Anxiety can almost always be handled by talking about it. Discussion helps to identify the true sources of anxiety and place reasonable bounds on it. Fears that can be communicated can be managed because words "contain" them.

When a fistula is suspected, it is accepted practice to first thoroughly evaluate the full extent of the problem prior to proceeding with treatment. In the same fashion, when it is suspected that anxiety is becoming an obstacle to dental care, the professional will usually want to encourage the patient to talk about it: "You seem uneasy," for example, or "You look a little nervous about the procedure."

Once the patient responds by trying to articulate his or her feelings, the appropriate response from the dental professional is an empathic paraphrase, "Oh, I see you really are troubled about the extent of the surgery," or "Yes, you do seem upset about having to have a root canal." A good empathic response names both the emotion and its cause without being judgmental or denying the validity of the patient's feelings. It will often elicit further clarification from the patient. Some patients may not even be aware of the extent and real nature of their anxiety or how badly it is hindering communication until an empathic response helps them get their feelings under control. Anxiety is reduced when patients see that the dental professional cares about their feelings.

The most common mistake is attempting to reassure an anxious patient. "Everything will be 'okay,' you have nothing to be afraid of" communicates that the patient's feelings do not matter. Only the patient can place realistic bounds on his or her anxiety. When professionals offer reassurance, they are really attempting to control their own anxiety. It seldom works because it is the nervous patient who is making the professional uneasy, and reassurance shuts the door on any discussion that might solve the problem.

ANGER

Detection

People show their anger through tight and rigid faces and posture (Table 8–2). Their movements are quick and abrupt. They hit or slam things like books and doors. They stare with "looks that could kill." When they speak, the sentences tend to be short, loud, and declarative. They are derogatory, critical, sarcastic, demanding, and challenging. Questions are often a sign of anger.[3]

What is most commonly seen is not anger, but attempts to suppress or control aggressive impulses or channel them in socially acceptable ways. Because anger is seldom directly expressed, it is a dangerous emotion, consuming a great deal of energy to control and direct it.

Function

Anger is a natural response to frustration.[5] It occurs when the path to reaching an important goal is blocked or when an unexpected obstacle prevents satisfaction of an important need. Like anxiety, it is an emotion with survival value; it presses the individual into action. It is also both biologically and historically conditioned. A patient might overreact to having to wait or having caries diagnosed. There is usually something in such a patient's background, unrelated to dental experience, that will explain the overreaction. Perhaps the patient has arrived after waiting in line

TABLE 8–2. CHARACTERISTICS OF ANGER

Function	Detection	Dental Sources
Responds to frustration of needs	Rigidity Short, forceful movements Loud speech Questions Challenges	Cost Manipulation Exposed shortcomings Blocked communication

Communication Problems	Management
Suppression Displacement to innocent persons No follow-through Logical thought disrupted Inflexibility	*Do:* Empathically understand *Don't:* Ignore, become defensive, reassure, appease

at the bank or after feuding with his or her spouse. The learning process also influences how anger is expressed. Big people are often gentle because they have been told from childhood that they might hurt someone. Women typically express their anger indirectly because strong actions and emotions are "unladylike."

Dental Sources

Few patients want to go to the dentist. It is usually an unplanned disruption and a major frustration. It is the rare individual who budgets time or funds for dentistry. A visit interrupts the day's activities and costs money that may have been planned for a major purchase such as a color television or a vacation. Being made to wait, being left unattended, being "processed" as though the dentist's time were more valuable than the patient's, and being given unattractive or no treatment options frustrate the needs for dignity and self-esteem. Heavy demands on dentists make frustration almost inevitable and thus anger is a commonly observed emotion among dental professionals.

Dentists tend to seriously underestimate how much anger patients feel.[6] Most of the anger is hidden because dentists, and to some extent their staffs, represent power and authority. A lesson learned early in life is not to antagonize those who could do you harm, especially while in a defenseless position.

Anger can be so thoroughly suppressed that it is denied or not recognized. It tends to be directed away from powerful people, even when they are the source of frustration. Auxiliaries might be blamed for the rough and unsympathetic treatment of an overbearing dentist. Anger might be directed toward inanimate objects ("This headgear never works") or routines ("Do I really have to wait 30 minutes before driving home?"). Or anger might be directed inward ("I'm just dumb. I can't seem to get anything you're saying"). In its extreme form, inwardly directed anger can be self-destructive, as in the patient who sabotages a surgical treatment by prematurely removing dressings or eating hard foods. A frequent form of hidden aggression is the question directed at the professional's dignity: "Do you really enjoy looking in all these dirty mouths day after day?" or "What are all those diplomas on the wall?" Hidden anger is such a common emotion in dentistry that it should be suspected whenever a patient's words or behavior fail to make sense.

Communication Problems

Anger, expressed or hidden, profoundly disrupts communication.[5] Logical thought and behavior are impaired; alternatives cannot be weighed impartially. Anger, like anxiety, constricts the focus of attention, and patients tend not to see or hear anything outside their concern. Anger also causes inflexibility. A dentist who cannot get an assistant to follow office routine will redouble efforts at forcing compliance. The longer the problem continues, the stronger the pressure, the less creative the alternatives considered, and the less likely that the dentist will alter the strategy. Anger is also a problem because it undermines the mutual respect upon which the treatment alliance is based and because it may provoke angry responses from dental professionals.

Management

Anger in the dental situation cannot be counted on to remain under cover. It will either build and erupt in a vocal form or it will erode rapport and take the form of complaints to family and friends about the insensitivities in the dental office. Because anger is bound to surface, it is wise to bring it out under controlled circumstances.

Hidden anger is handled like anxiety. When it is suspected, the patient or co-worker is invited to discuss it. The response is answered with empathic understanding. If the source can be located it may be corrected.

When a patient's anger is directed at the dentist or the staff, it is particularly hard to handle. Even when ostensibly aimed at the professional, the source of anger may be elsewhere and there is no need to become defensive. Complaints about fees might stem from failure of the patient's company to provide dental insurance. Bitterness over unexpected treatment might be partially the result of fatigue and stress on the job. When the dental professional is entirely responsible for the anger, it is best to admit so openly and make appropriate changes. It is easier to stay mad at a "self-righteous, insensitive, incompetent person" than one who "makes an honest mistake."

Handling open, verbal anger requires considerable skill. It is made easier by recognizing two important things about the actively angry individual: they are typically vulnerable and afraid and they need to have their anger recognized. Abusive, antagonistic, and vocally aggressive patients have such strong needs that they are willing to risk social disapproval in order to call their emotions to someone's attention. Such strong feelings can usually be defused by repeatedly paraphrasing the angry person's feelings in a nonjudgmental fashion. Anger will persist until someone says, "Yes, I see your anger and it is legitimate to be angry for the reasons you have." For example, "With all those expenses at home, I can see why you're upset about needing a root canal."

There are three common mistakes made in dealing with anger. Attempting to ignore the situation has already been mentioned as ineffective. Defensiveness merely escalates anger in a cyclical fashion. "I resent that kind of remark" precipitates a shouting match or loses a patient or a co-worker. Perhaps the most common trap is appeasement. "Yes, Mr. Bumbry, we'll get to you right away. I'm doing everything possible." These individuals have not had their anger recognized as being legitimate: they have been put down. The unspoken words that accompany appeasement are "I don't know what's upsetting you but I'll give you something just to get you off my back."

DEPRESSION

Detection

Depression shows in persons who lack normal responsiveness in voice, facial expression, and posture (Table 8–3). Compared with facial expression, posture is a particularly reliable indicator because it is not as consciously controlled. The "weight of the world" can be seen in drooping shoulders, a "ponch" in the abdomen, and slouching when sitting. Persons who are depressed appear preoccupied with themselves, especially their feelings. They are apt to use words like "down," "can't get started," or "can't do anything right." They apologize frequently. They are likely to cry and unlikely to follow through on suggestions or commitments.[3]

TABLE 8–3. CHARACTERISTICS OF DEPRESSION

Function	Detection	Dental Sources
Reaction to loss, particularly self-esteem	Sagging posture Unresponsiveness Talk of own worthlessness Lack of emotional control	Diagnosis that work is needed Disappointment with self, child, or past dentistry

Communication Problems	Management
Distraction Lack of self-confidence No motivation for follow-through	*Do:* Give explicit instructions and much feedback; determine nature of problem, delay giving directions *Don't:* Force commitment

Function

Depression is the emotional reaction to loss or unexpected defeat.[7] Although the loss may be physical, depression is frequently the result of a blow to one's self-esteem or self-image. Mild depression is common and it affects most of us at one time or another. It tends to resolve itself in a short time and is not dangerous, even though it may complicate communication and dental treatment. On the other hand, severe depression, which persists and involves contemplation of bodily injury, is cause for concern and requires professional help.

Dental Sources

Unlike anxiety and anger, which arise and subside quickly, depression may last for days or weeks. Most of the depression seen in dental offices is unrelated to the dental situation, although some exceptions exist. A diagnosis that dental work is needed can be a blow to one's ego, particularly if the therapy is protracted. Parents can become depressed over their children's needed care.

Communication Problems

Regardless of the source, depressed patients lack the self-confidence and enthusiasm to make decisions or to follow through on suggestions. They hear the postsurgical instructions, but they are just too much for them to handle. Planning treatment and arranging a payment schedule may be frustrating or ineffective.

Management

No drastic intervention is called for in the case of mildly depressed patients. It is wise to engage in discussion sufficient to determine whether the depression is dentally related. Depressed patients are easy to talk to. They do not mind a sympathetic audience when they rehearse their injuries, slights, injustices, and shortcomings. Extra time and care are required in giving instructions and, if possible, major decisions and commitments should be postponed until the depression resolves itself. If depression continues over several appointments and appears to interfere with normal functions, it would be appropriate to ask the patient or co-worker whether professional care has been considered.

Patients who cry in the dental office present an awkward problem. They usually embarrass the dentist and the staff, and no one knows exactly what to do. The natural tendency is to offer support and reassurance while saying either "Now, now; there's no need to cry" or "That's 'okay.' Go ahead and cry if you feel like it."

This may shorten the crying, but it also cuts short the emotional release and may make the patient feel ashamed. The recommended response is to wait quietly and attentively until the patient stops crying. An empathic response may be added, "You must be very upset," to encourage them to talk. Sometimes patients are choked with emotion and cannot communicate effectively. The dental professional can help clear this obstruction by suggesting, "You look like you are so sad you could cry."

APATHY

Detection

Those whose cheerfulness is shallow, stiff, and forced or who have a vacant look and are slow to respond might be suspected of being apathetic (Table 8–4). The posture and lack of enthusiasm in apathy are similar to what is seen in depression. The critical difference is the way individuals talk about their emotions.[7] Depressed patients are preoccupied by their moods. Apathetic people avoid mentioning their own or anyone's emotions and will often deny that they have feelings. They appear overly cooperative and say "Oh, I don't care," "If you say so . . . ," or "Whatever you think," but as soon as the structure provided by the dental professional is removed, the apathetic patient is incapable of sustaining the behavior to which they have agreed.

Function

Apathy is an effort to deny or destroy all emotions.[1] It is a vital protective device similar to a circuit breaker that temporarily shuts

TABLE 8–4. CHARACTERISTICS OF APATHY

Function	Detection	Dental Sources
Turning-off of emotions to protect from overload	Stiff Expressionless Unresponsive Avoidance of talking about problems	Surgery Extensive restorations Life-threatening diseases

Communication Problems	Management
Inability to concentrate Lack of motivation Desire to escape and avoid	*Do:* Delay explanations, provide written instructions, involve relatives *Don't:* Describe situation as hopeless

off all emotional equipment when there is an overload. Assistants who work for overbearing dentists, for example, control their vulnerable feelings by hiding them until the danger is past. Becoming emotionally invisible is a natural response to both physical and psychological threats and is frequently seen in victims of persecution, discrimination, or chauvinism. Apathy tends to last as long as the defense is needed. When the threat passes or when sufficient coping strength is marshaled, apathy resolves itself.

Dental Sources

The most common causes of apathy in dentistry are surgery and chronic degenerative conditions such as oral cancer or severe periodontical involvement. Fear and anger are strong emotions compounded by a helplessness and sense of inevitability. Few patients can continue to face the prospect of pain and disfiguration for any period of time. The alternative is to paralyze the emotions. "I don't care about my teeth. Take them all out." Auxiliaries are often apathetic in response to a sense of inescapable inferiority in their jobs.

Communication Problems

Apathy may actually be beneficial in cases such as surgery. Some people can reduce the physical sensations of pain and become semi-comatose. But before and afterward it will cause complications. Postsurgical instructions may be entirely missed. The patient might nod agreement throughout and telephone that evening to ask about things that have been thoroughly covered. When apathy lasts longer than a few hours it can impair patients' recuperative responses. Patients who have killed all their emotions have also killed hope and the will to heal themselves. Immediate denture treatment can fail because of an apathetic response. In less extreme cases, patients who receive bad news about their oral health may become apathetic about taking any responsibility for correcting the problem. Large and prolonged treatments may be just too much for some patients to handle emotionally.

Management

Dental professionals should avoid creating apathy among patients. No situation should be described as more hopeless than it is. Scare tactics should be avoided. A very fine line must be walked between giving false hope in serious problems and stressing the futility of the situation.[2]

When treating patients who are apathetic, some precautions must be observed. It is advisable to write down key instructions and to have a friend or relative present during treatment planning and post-treatment conversations. It is also suggested that the dentist should telephone such patients to check on progress and reiterate important instructions. In cases of severe apathy, it helps to get patients involved. Surgical cases may require following a special diet and instructions for caring for the surgical site. Such patients may be advised to telephone the office to give periodic progress reports.

IMPATIENCE

Detection

Some patients or co-workers sit with their hands on the edge of the seat; they drum their fingers and swing their feet; place their hands on their hips or the arm of the chair as if they are ready to leave; and they fix a questioning gaze on something or someone. These people are impatient and they are signaling that they are ready for something to happen (Table 8–5). They manage to make others uncomfortable. When things go too far for them, they interrupt or hurry the conversation on to its conclusion, "Yes, yes, I know" or "So . . .?"[8] Such impatient interrupting is called "pseudoagreement."

Function

Impatience is a natural protective reaction. Impatient individuals are defending themselves from information and emotional over-

TABLE 8–5. CHARACTERISTICS OF IMPATIENCE

Function	Detection	Dental Sources
Protection from overload	"Forward" posture Repetitive, rythmic movements Fixed gaze Interruptions "Pseudoagreement"	Too much information Long appointments Waiting Lack of control over situation

Communication Problems	Management
Avoidance of responsibility Difficulty in listening Anger	*Do:* Structure time, provide activity, monitor nonverbals *Don't:* Explain in detail, avoid excessive rationality

load.[9] They are stressed and they avoid absorbing any more external stimulation by pressing for any action that promises to reduce stress. The famous quotation "My mind is made up, don't confuse me with facts" suits them. "Getting on with the work at hand" is also a substitute for considering their own or others' feelings. Impatient people often see emotions as a trap that requires their energy and threatens their sense of control because it is uncertain where a discussion on the emotional level might lead.

Dental Sources

The cause of impatience is conflicting pressures under stress. Dentists themselves are more apt to experience this emotion than are patients or auxiliaries. Sometimes patients may feel pressured by tediously thorough examinations, complex treatment plans, ambiguous diagnoses, ambivalent prognoses, and delayed appointments. Patients who are already late, preoccupied by domestic or other cares, or place dental care low on their hierarchy of concerns are apt to find optimal dental care to be tiresome. To such patients, even the courtesies of a friendly staff are resented as a waste of time. Such patients want to be told what must be done and then to have it completed with the least amount of fuss and delay possible.

Communication Problems

It may appear that individuals who agree with almost anything and value swift service are ideal patients. They are not. They are unlikely to accept personal responsibility for their own care and generally endure post-visit instruction or preventive messages only as long as is necessary to finish the appointment. Their apparent ready agreement is a strategy for avoiding lengthy discussions. Impatient patients will skimp on their medical histories and avoid elaborating on any comment, including their chief complaint. An ever-present problem with impatient individuals is the danger that they will become angry.

Impatient dentists are often surprised by the unexpected behavior of patients and staff because these dentists have assumed more than they have communicated. They demand structure, organization, efficiency, and people around them who are talented enough to read their minds or submissive enough to accept responsibility for existing miscommunication. They are unlikely to have read this far in this text.

Management
Impatient individuals need structure and action to reduce their stress. They should be told what is being done at each moment and what activities will follow. Nonverbal clues as to how an impatient person is handling the provided structure must be continually monitored and are usually more effective than verbal interactions. It does little good to reason with an impatient person.[10] They do not want to hear why more information is necessary or why a procedure takes so long. The patient sees this as further delay and more useless information. Decisions that are made by impatient individuals should be confirmed later when pressures are lessened. Signs of impatience must be carefully observed during persuasion. They are a signal to avoid overselling.

COMMUNICATING THE PROFESSIONALS' EMOTIONS

Dentists and staff experience anxiety, anger, depression, apathy, and impatience just as patients do, and these emotions stem from similar sources and serve the same protective functions.[11] What differs is the way professionals are expected to express their feelings.

Although it is acceptable to let a patient know how upset you are that a piece of lab work is late or that you just broke an instrument on the bench, this is done primarily to inform. Care is taken to avoid any impression that the professional is not in control, that the patient is supposed to help the professional, or that reflects negatively on any part of the health care team. It is expected that all emotions originating outside the office will not become overt in the office and that all intraoffice emotional tension will be managed so as not to affect patient care. Chapter 16 addresses this matter in detail.

When the patient is the source of the emotion, the situation should be handled assertively. Emotions are contagious. Empathic and assertive responses help the professional manage strong feelings that otherwise potentially can disrupt objectivity and care.

- *(Hygienist to patient)* "You know, I really feel cheated because I worked so hard to restore your gums to health and you promised you would take care of them like we discussed. And now look. You haven't flossed in two weeks." (Communicates anger without prompting defensiveness)

Occasionally patients or staff members have emotional problems that are beyond their control. In such cases referral is indicated, and the techniques described in this chapter are only a necessary first step: they disclose the existence and something of the magnitude of the problem. The second step involves messages such as the following:

- "This appears to be a problem that will require modifying what I had planned for today. It isn't right to ask you to make a decision when you are so upset."
- "I'm sorry, Mr. Thomas, but I can't function safely or effectively when you have these emotional outbursts. As the situation doesn't seem to be getting any better, I think we need to recognize it as a problem and talk about some of the things you can do."
- "Martha, I'm worried about you. You haven't been yourself. You're forgetful about your medication and your mouth shows that you haven't been taking care of yourself. Because I am concerned, I'm going to ask you whether you have sought any professional counseling since Jack died."

CASE: RESPONDING TO THE RIGHT EMOTION

A patient-of-record with no appointment, a businessman, recoiled from the front desk and slapped his hands on the counter. Then he tensed up and leaned forward.

Patient: "What do you mean, 'the Doctor doesn't have any openings this afternoon'?"

Receptionist: "I know it's frustrating for you not to be able to see Dr. Minsky when you've taken time out to come to the office."

Patient: "Is that all you can say, how frustrated I must be? I tell you, all doctors are alike—so high and mighty"

Receptionist: "You seem to be annoyed because you think that Dr. Minsky doesn't care about you."

Patient: "What does he care. He has a room full of patients waiting. My internist is worse. I have persistent stomach problems and I can't even get in to see him for two weeks. And my accountant! You want to hear a hot one? I've got buyers lined up for my business and he is out of town on a vacation. It seems like you've got to be 'somebody' before anybody pays attention to you. I've got more problems than your Dr. Minsky ever dreamed of."

Receptionist: "You sound like a very busy man. Let's see if there's anything I can do with the appointment book for later this week."

Patient: "You bet I'm busy. I don't have time for these problems. When can I get to see the doctor?"

Receptionist: "It looks like we have two choices. I can get you in as an emergency at eleven on Tuesday, or Thursday morning is 'okay' if you don't mind coming in at 8:30. The choice is yours."

Patient: "Well, like I say, I'm awfully busy. So give me the 8:30 on Thursday. And by the way, Dr. Minsky doesn't realize how lucky he is to have someone on the ball like you covering the front desk for him."

The receptionist records the appointment and places a note in the patient's chart explaining the circumstances and asking Dr. Minsky to speak with the patient about the importance of advanced planning.

ANALYSIS

This one-minute encounter is complex, and it was handled tactfully and effectively by the receptionist. The receptionist actually begins by responding to the wrong emotion, anger. The questioning, sharp and conspicuous body movements, and aggressive posture are all symptomatic of anger and the receptionist's empathic reflection of this mood is appropriate for such a feeling. Two such empathic responses are used to draw out the fact that the patient seems to resent authority in general and is specifically mad at two other professionals. The fundamental emotion, impatience, is uncovered. The receptionist manages the patient by first letting him know that she sees his impatience and then by very specific actions and involvement of the patient. In a very few words, the receptionist has diagnosed a complex emotion and saved a patient for the practice, while avoiding a potentially embarrassing confrontation.

Patients' emotions are not always easily categorized. In this case impatience was masked by anger, a common defensive posture. The receptionist's first empathic response actually provoked sarcasm because it addressed and perhaps aggravated a symptom rather than addressing the source of the problem. The receptionist was still right in the strategy taken. It would have been a guess to go right for a structured solution with the appointment book, and the resolution would have been more superficial. The moral is that managing emotions requires more listening than talking, and faith in both yourself and others.

REFERENCES

1. Brammer, L.E., & Shostrom, E.L. *Therapeutic psychology: Fundamentals of counseling and psychotherapy* (3rd. ed.). Englewood Cliffs, New Jersey: Prentice-Hall, 1977.
2. Chambers, D.W. Coping with stress. In S.S. Boundy & N.J. Reynolds, (Eds.), *Current concepts in dental hygiene* (vol. 3.). St Louis: C.V. Mosby, 1979, pp. 155–168.
3. Froelich, R.E., Bishop, F.M., & Dworkin, S.F. *Communication in the dental office: A programmed manual for the dental professional.* St Louis: C.V. Mosby, 1976.
4. Selye, H. *The stress of life.* New York: McGraw-Hill, 1956.
5. Lazarus, R.S. *Psychological stress and the coping process.* New York: McGraw-Hill, 1966.
6. Dworkin, S.F, Ference, T.P., & Giddon, D.B. *Behavioral science and dental practice.* St Louis: C.V. Mosby, 1978.
7. Bird, B.: *Talking with patients* (2nd. ed.). Philadelphia: J.B. Lippincott, 1973.
8. Knapp, M.L. *Nonverbal communication in human interaction* (2nd ed.). New York: Holt, Rinehart and Winston, 1978.
9. Miller, J.G. Information input overload. In M.C. Yovits, G.T. Jacobi, and G.D. Goldstein (Eds.), *Self-regulating systems.* Washington, D.C.: Spartan, 1962.
10. Festinger, L. *A theory of cognitive dissonance.* Stanford, Calif.: Stanford University Press, 1957.
11. Viscott, D. *The language of feelings.* New York: Pocket Books, 1976.

EXERCISES

8–1. Match the symptoms below with their probable emotions:

- **a.** Gazing past the speaker, slouching, responding slowly, and denying that anything is wrong when questioned.
- **b.** Looking down distractedly at one's hands, hunching over, speaking softly, and repeating how tired one is and how unfair the world is.
- **c.** Staring at an object on the desk, sitting erect, and agreeing too quickly with the speaker.
- **d.** Eyes darting from object to object, not knowing where to start a sentence, repeating oneself, and answering direct questions with "I'm not sure."

8–2. Practice active listening skills in an emotional context. Practice switching your focus away from what a person is saying to the context (why should they be saying this now?), the status (who do they think I am that they should speak like this to me?), and the nonverbals (how are they expressing themselves?).

8–3. List management considerations for the following patient. What would you want to do and what would you avoid doing?

> You are describing the relationship between plaque and dental disease and presenting the benefits that can be gained from the patient's participating in your three-session oral hygiene program. The patient nods in general agreement, but occasionally agrees with statements like "and you don't want to feed the bacteria . . ." which should elicit a negative response. He seems bored and complains of being tired today. Once when you ask him a direct question he apologizes, "Oh, I'm sorry. I must have been thinking of something else."

8–4. Try role playing with a friend. Have your partner pretend to be justifiably angry at something you are supposed to have done. First try defusing the anger by accepting responsibility and reflecting empathy with your friend's feelings. Now do it again, but this time justify yourself and reflect back the hurt and anger you feel.

DISCUSSION OF EXERCISES

8–1. The nonverbal clues in the first two cases show people who have been defeated by the world. Apathy, the first example, can be distinguished from depression, the second example, by the former patient's unwillingness to talk about emotions. The erect posture in Example 3 suggests a more active emotion such as anger or impatience. Avoiding eye contact and pseudoagreement that cuts off others' speech are more representative of impatience. The fourth example is of anxiety, showing several instances of inability to concentrate and loss of control without any sign of aggression. Hidden anger is also a possibility.

8–2. By using all the channels available for listening and by evaluating their consistency, it should be possible to learn more and learn more quickly about others' feelings. It is also important to treat perceived emotions as hypotheses in active listening. You might want to verify your perceptions ("You really seem down today") before you attempt to manage the emotion.

8–3. This patient exhibits many of the symptoms of depression—or perhaps apathy. A persuasive message about oral hygiene would likely be ineffective; in fact it might damage later attempts to motivate this patient. A few questions should be asked to determine the extent of the depression and whether it has a dental origin. Postpone seeking a commitment because the depression will probably have resolved itself the next time you see the patient. You will both feel better if you do not press the issue.

8–4. It is not important to be polished in this exercise. What you should experience is some uneasiness on the part of both persons when reflecting empathy, but the angry actor will generally find it difficult to continue even pretending to be angry. When anger is reflected back it should generate an escalating spiral of emotion, one which is easier to sustain but does not lead to a satisfactory resolution.

9

Children and Older Patients

Dealing with children and older patients requires special communication skills. The complex and at times disorderly changes that occur in the mouth of the young and the elderly are matched by developmental trends in their intellectual and emotional lives. Treating them without regard for these underlying dynamics results in less than optimal care.

Although diversity and variability are characteristic of such patients, there are two consistent themes that are of value:

- It is wise to assume that the behavior and language of children and older patients are meaningful and perfectly natural *to them* even when they may appear inconsistent, illogical, or unexpected.[1]
- The emotional aspects of communication often predominate in what these patients and their families say. Literal focus on the information component of messages can be misleading.[2]

A convenient way of displaying the full array of intellectual and emotional diversity in these patients will be to describe the central theme and behavior of each age group. Management do's and don't's for health professionals are then suggested. Six groups are presented: (1) toddlers, (2) preschoolers, (3) young children, (4) preadolescents, (5) adolescents, and (6) older persons. Finally, some comments are made about the families of these special patients.

Often age divisions between the groups are not precise because people mature at different rates and great variations can be seen. The generalizations offered here should afford a useful way to see the special worlds of these patients. By recognizing the differences, the dental professional will be better able to communicate and respond to the needs of children and older patients.[3]

TODDLERS (ROUGHLY 12 TO 36 MONTHS)

Theme and Behavior

Children between 1 and 3 years of age are learning about the world of other people and the limits of their own will.[4] A major source of frustration for them is the inability to express themselves completely in words. "No" is the central word in the toddler's life, used to indicate what is dangerous and unacceptable. "Mine" is also important because the outside world and everything that is not "mine" can be threatening. It is understandable that the toddler's reaction to strangers is unpredictable. These two words place limits on children's activity and are the origin of their self-concept (Table 9–1).

Management

Toddlers are typically treated with the parent present, often holding the child on his or her lap. Some 2-year-olds will sit in the dental chair and permit an oral examination. Most of the verbal communication is between the dentist and the parent, but this relationship is watched carefully by the child. Communication with the child typically is nonverbal and indirect. Quiet, soft, and reassuring voice and movements are important. The "fear of strangers" reaction can be triggered by sudden movements or loud commands—toward the child or the parent. Prolonged staring or sudden reaching for the child are not recommended. Rapport with the parent is the key to successful communication with the toddler.

TABLE 9–1. CHARACTERISTICS OF TODDLERS

Characteristics	Professional Response
Self-expression frustrated	Use calm, slow, reassuring language and gestures
Learning limits of own freedom	
Reactions to strangers unpredictable	Develop rapport with parent

The child reads and reflects his or her reactions to the professional. Inability to communicate may not necessarily reflect on dental professionals' lack of communication skills. Even with the most skillful approach, the 2-year-old may scream and cry during an examination, preventing any real communication.

PRESCHOOL (ROUGHLY 3 TO 5 YEARS)

Theme and Behavior

Children in this age group have discovered the outside world of physical objects but they are struggling to learn how they relate to it. This leads to a jumble of inconsistent behavior and strange language that is both amusing and frustrating (Table 9–2).[4]

Management

Preschoolers interpret adult speech literally. If a dentist is overheard complaining about advice that falls on cold ears, the typical 5-year-old may want to feel the ears in question to see how cold they are. The same child may shy away from the receptionist who says, "How cute you are, I could just eat you up." "Substitute phrases" must be carefully chosen, such as those in Table 9–3. If a child is told that you are going to "look at his teeth," he or she does not expect you to touch them. Children who are fearful of going to sleep may not appreciate being told that you are going to "put their tooth to sleep." Use simple words, short sentences, and talk slowly.

Inanimate objects are often invested with feelings and other signs of life. A broken bicycle is "hurt." Noisy machinery is "angry." Dental equipment may appear menacing. It is predictable that the hissing, spitting, whining handpiece is alive, scary, and apparently quite angry.

TABLE 9–2. CHARACTERISTICS OF PRESCHOOLERS

Characteristics	Professional Response
Interpret language literally	Avoid metaphors
Invest inanimate objects with feelings	Explain equipment in nonthreatening way
Color perceptions with feelings	Suggest appropriate interpretations, avoid nonverbal expressions of anxiety
Imprecise concept of sensations	Avoid logic
Lack reasoning skills	Set acceptable rules for behavior
Inconsistent and forgetful	

TABLE 9–3. EXAMPLES OF SUBSTITUTE DENTAL TERMINOLOGY FOR YOUNG CHILDREN

Dental Term	Substitute Word
Air syringe	Wind, air
Alginate material	Pudding, dough
Anesthetic	Sleepy tooth medicine, juice
Burr	Brush
Dental caries	Brown spot, sick tooth
Explorer	Tooth feeler, counter
Fluoride	Tooth toughener, vitamins
Hand piece	Hose, tooth cleaner, water whistle
High speed evacuator	Vacuum cleaner
Pit and fissure sealant	Plastic cover, clean tooth polish
Rubber dam	Rubber raincoat
Stainless steel crown	Hat for tooth
Study models	Statues
X-ray equipment	Tooth camera
X-ray film	Tooth picture

Preschoolers' perceptions of the world are colored by their values, and size can be confused with importance. A toy a child wants is literally seen as larger than an unattractive toy of the same size.[5] All adults are large, but threatening ones are enormous. Instruments that are sharp may loom in frightening proportions. The space left by a lost tooth may appear very large. Explaining the significance and use of dental equipment in nonthreatening terms is helpful in reducing the chances that such equipment may be seen as dangerous by preschoolers. The common management technique of "tell–show–do" can be used to minimize fear. For example, after describing the handpiece as a noisy water hose, one can demonstrate in the dentist's and then the child's hand how it sprays water and will wash the tooth.

Children of this age are also learning about bodily sensations.[6] Nitrous oxide or local injections will be labeled pleasant, awkward, uncomfortable, or terrifying by the child depending on how they are explained by the dental professional and the child's family. A tense face, quick movements, and a little wince are all children need to convince them that they are supposed to feel uncomfortable. The professional can also verbally help young children learn about their sensations. When giving an injection, the dentist may suggest, "You will feel a little pinch but it will just last a short time" or, following the initial needle penetration, "It will feel like a balloon filling up."

Children aged 3 to 5 or 6 years also lack the reasoning ability necessary to make promises, compare present to future actions, or understand analogies. Reasoning with preschoolers may give the impression of success if the children are sensitive enough to know when they are supposed to say "yes." It is the nonverbal communication and not the logic that really controls the child's behavior.[7]

Adults use the question as a form of polite suggestion. To the literal-minded child "would you like to get into the chair now?" is an invitation to answer truthfully, "No." It is wise to avoid giving children unrealistic or undesirable choices. A preferable phrasing is, "It is time to get into the chair now."[8]

Preschool children are active, expressive, and forgetful. A child who is squirming, fidgeting, and in need of constant reminders is not necessarily disobedient. The 4- or 5-year-old does not live in the same logical, consistent, and objective world that the dentist and the dental staff live in. It is a waste of time to demand that they try to do so. Most preschoolers require continued correction, prompting, and some physical control. The experts in handling such children do not expect them to behave like adults and, when necessary, do not hesitate to use behavior management techniques that are not based on communication.[9]

YOUNG CHILD (ROUGHLY 5 TO 7 OR 8 YEARS)

Theme and Behavior

The young child is proud and vulnerable.[4] Children who are 5 to 7 or 8 years old have a new pride in themselves, their body and possessions. They will talk endlessly about how big they are or what new clothes and toys they have. This appearance of bravery and maturity is also a hopeful facade that is easily pierced. Young children are concerned over self-control. When apprehensive 6-year-olds display a fear of dentistry, they are embarrassed and humiliated. Dental professionals may appeal to the child's wanting to be mature but should avoid undermining a young child's confidence (Table 9–4).

Management

Finding the right balance of confidence, while remaining believable and avoiding ridicule, is difficult. The three sentences below

TABLE 9–4. CHARACTERISTICS OF YOUNG CHILDREN

Characteristics	Professional Response
Pride in accomplishments and ownership	Appeal to maturity, solicit child's help
Vulnerable to loss of face and self-control	Avoid embarrassment
Concern over body	Care and sensitivity during examination and injection
	Give child some control

differ only slightly, yet each may affect a young patient in different ways.

- "Grown up boys and girls usually remain very still, and I know you can do it too." (Appeal to pride)
- "I can tell you're a big, brave girl who never moves around in the chair." (Universals such as "never" and superfluous qualification such as "big, brave" reduce credibility)
- "I don't want you to squirm around like your little sister." (The comparison with a younger child is damaging to the young patient's pride.)

A special source of embarrassment among young children is crying in the dental office. There is no scientific evidence that crying is harmful to the child. It is a normal release of strong emotions magnified in a fearful situation. In fact, there are reports in the medical literature of children passively enduring injections and later in the day developing violent reactions such as rashes, vomiting, nightmares, and enuresis.[2]

The problem with crying is distinguishing the normal release of emotion from tantrums that are used to control adults and to postpone treatment. Tantrums should be controlled with behavior management techniques.[7] Emotional crying should be handled exactly as an adult who showed strong feelings would be handled—with patience and empathy: "I can see you're unhappy or afraid, but I'll try to explain everything to you."

The pride young people take in their bodies can make them unusually sensitive to bodily harm. The smallest cut may be elaborated into a mortal wound. Confining illnesses during this time can lead to personality damage.[2] It is no wonder that dentists who drill holes, cut, and extract are viewed with great alarm. They violate the young child's fragile but important self-concept. The professional's support is particularly helpful in such cases as extractions: "I know you're unhappy about losing the baby tooth, but soon you will have new grown up teeth like your friends" or ". . . the Tooth Fairy will be looking for it."

Preoccupation with pride and control make two parts of dental care particularly anxiety-provoking. The examination, which patients of other ages appear to tolerate, is frightening to young children. They are afraid that the dentist will pierce their protective shield. Warts, cheek biting, and blisters can be sources of concern. Dental equipment like vitality testers and the radiographic unit have magical and dangerous powers. The other difficult part of the procedure is anesthesia. This is a test of their self-control. General anesthesia is particularly challenging. Sleep represents loss of control. Often these children are afraid that the dentist will do something to them while they are asleep or that they will talk in their sleep or fail to control their bladder. At such times it is helpful to give children some degree of control. For example, when given an injection they may be invited to raise their hand if there is some problem.

Young children are changeable, from cooperation to obstruction to withdrawal to excitement. It is probably more accurate to say that they are testing themselves rather than the dental professional. Anyone who can help a child master a difficult situation will be on the way toward having a cooperative patient. First, the professional must respect the child's needs and limits. Children should not be lied to or misled. Their help can be enlisted in holding equipment or a mirror. Recall and appointment reminders can be mailed directly to the young patient.

PREADOLESCENTS (ROUGHLY 8 YEARS OLD TO PUBERTY)

Theme and Behavior

Prior to puberty, children are concerned with the outside world of things and people and how they fit into it.[10] They approach these problems through mental operations and language, which are growing during this period. Preadolescents sound grown up, but their grasp of adult language is fragmentary and inconsistent.

These children are likely to say the strangest things.[4] Their conversation may jump from one topic to another and frequently takes the form of questions. "Why does your nurse have a blue dress and everybody else is in white?" "Mommy wrecked the car today, gee!" "If somebody kills somebody will they have to go to jail?" Their language is cryptic and symbolic and often has double meanings. Dental professionals must work especially hard at listening for meaning and avoid taking preadolescent's language literally. On the other hand, if their language is unclear, it still may be significant. The question about the uniform's color may be a way of finding out about status and the qualifications of the hygienist. The question about jail may express concern over something the child has done or fear about the dentist's skill (Table 9–5).

Management

Preadolescents typically present fewer behavior problems than younger children and consequently receive less attention from adults. Dental professionals must assume that there is more going on with preadolescents than meets the eye and they should participate in their patients' communication, even when it is seemingly without purpose. "Oh, your sister lost her bicycle. What did she do? What do you think about that?"

The preadolescent's world is a strange jumble of the literal and the imaginary. They may feel that fluoride toothpaste colors the inside of teeth, that food rots teeth, that all old people have dentures like Grandpa, that policemen will arrest children who fail to brush their teeth, or that their new permanent teeth will fall out just as their baby ones did. Such children will benefit from careful and concrete explanations of everything the dental professional does.

One of the dangers in communicating with children of this age is the adult's overestimation of the child's mental capacity. In this age group, use of language significantly exceeds intellectual ability. They may be able to talk about "plaque," "caries," or "hygiene" with great conviction and at the proper time. Yet their understanding of these words will be blurred, imprecise, or even absent. Preadolescents exhibit a wide range of ability to weigh future and present benefits, to see the consequences of hypothetical courses of

TABLE 9–5. CHARACTERISTICS OF PREADOLESCENTS

Characteristics	Professional Response
Cryptic, symbolic language Jumping from topic to topic	Listen for meaning, not literal interpretation
Mixture of literal and imaginary concepts	Treat all questions seriously, provide full explanations
Appears to understand more than really comprehended	Do not assume child knows what he or she can talk about

action, to accept responsibility for the results of their behavior, to compare dissimilar alternatives, and to adopt another's point of view. Acquiring these intellectual skills is not a smooth and consistent process. Preadolescents lack the capacity for reasoning by analogy and being objective. The dental professional who reasons with preadolescents will be frustrated by the inconsistencies of these children who "talk a better game than they can deliver."

ADOLESCENTS

Theme and Behavior

Teenagers are making the transition from childhood to being adults. The shift from the absorbing subjectivity of childhood to an objective, logical view of the grown-up world is completed during these years. The major problem confronting teenagers is their emotional development, which incorporates the volatile characteristics of idealism, inconsistency, projection, and hero-worship.[11] This is the time to establish a personal identity, which is accomplished by trying on a variety of roles and world views in rapid succession or even simultaneously (Table 9–6).[1]

Management

It is important that the dental professional represent a clear and consistent image so as not to further confuse the adolescent patient.[12] Reasonable limits are proper for punctuality, oral hygiene, and conformance with orthodontic homecare regimens and these are generally appreciated.

The special vocabulary of teenagers can be a communication problem. Current lingo changes with great rapidity and frustrates the best attempts of adults to remain up-to-date. Confusing outsiders is an important part of this vocabulary, which serves for group identification and to define status.[13] The best strategy is to listen

TABLE 9–6. CHARACTERISTICS OF ADOLESCENTS

Characteristics	Professional Response
Uneven emotional development	Set reasonable limits and standards
Constantly changing over-identification with different models	Respond in standard English
	Honestly express your feelings
Argot (private language)	
Noncommunicative periods	

and attempt to understand the adolescent, but to respond in consistent standard English.

Teenagers can also be noncommunicative. At times they give a minimal civil response, answer "Who knows?", or just shrug their shoulders. These inarticulate periods may stem from confusion over roles; they will pass with time. It is unwise for the dental professional to try to relate to teenagers on "their" terms—the ground rules change too quickly. Honestly expressed frustration over the breakdown in communication is more effective.

- "It really bothers me when you don't pay attention."
- "When I have to repeat myself, I get upset."

OLDER PATIENTS

Theme and Behavior

Communication with older patients is complicated by declining physical and mental capacity and by their relative lack of concern for social convention.[2] Partial loss of sight, hearing, sensation, and memory may be unrecognized by the patient, or they may try to hide these from the dentist. Concern over loss of capacity increases the need for personal respect, attention, and dignity. The attitudes and behaviors of the elderly may indicate a disregard for social mores and conduct (Table 9–7).

Management

Older patients require and appreciate clear and straightforward explanations. Frequent repetition or written directions are often required. New behaviors or practices may be difficult to learn if they are contrary to the habits of a lifetime. Older persons are also more careless in observing social convention. "Don't worry about me, Dear. I know I should be brushing, but I'm old enough to do as

TABLE 9–7. CHARACTERISTICS OF OLDER PATIENTS

Characteristics	Professional Response
Diminished hearing, sight, memory, reasoning capacity	Simple, repeated explanations
Disregard for convention	Assertiveness not always effective
Concern over "care" aspect of treatment	Involvement of patient, discuss needs
Strong need for dignity	Acceptance of needs, to extent this does not compromise treatment

I please now." This makes the skills of persuasion and assertiveness, presented earlier in this text, less effective. It is not that I-messages and persuasion based on consistency between values and behavior is wrong, it is just not as likely to work with older patients. Oddly, most elderly people expect others to conform socially. They can be quite upset by any lapse of professionalism, such as the assistant not showing the "doctor" proper authority and respect.

Older patients are very concerned over health care, with more emphasis on *care* than on health. They can take great interest in the intricate details of treatment and they appreciate full explanations. Some older patients even use ailments that have no physical manifestations, such as denture discomfort, in order to secure sympathy and concern. When this becomes a problem, it should be addressed directly.

- "I can see that you are still bothered by that problem. But I have exhausted every means of dealing with it. Would you like to talk about it?"
- "Let's talk about what you expect from me in the way of care, Mrs. Daniels."

Of great significance to all older patients is their need for dignity. Society and advancing age have taken so much from older Americans that their sense of self-worth and respect becomes paramount. In some regards, they resemble young children in their concern for their body, their possessions, and their vulnerable pride. Dental health professionals should find ways for older patients to "be right" and participate without compromising their health or their pride.

- "Naturally, I will replace those crowns if that is what you want. I can see why you would want to look your best. There are some other options that will give the same results. Would you like to hear about them?"
- "I have a way of doing it, but first I'd like to see how you would go about cleaning this denture."

FAMILY

Parents and relatives provide the context in which communication with patients takes place. They help interpret, reinforce, negate, or alter what the dental professional says. They have helped to form part of the intellectual and emotional world in which the patient lives. At the same time, the family does not always have a positive influence on the patient and his or her dental care. Parents may feel guilty and defensive when their child has "a bad check up." Older patients and their spouses or children may try to play the dentist against each other. The unique needs of family members must be discerned and acknowledged.

Whenever a patient has a limitation of physical, intellectual, or emotional capacity, it is desirable to have family members present. This may include routine treatment of young children, the information-gathering and decision-making phases of treatment for any patient, and post-treatment or homecare instructions. The parent or family member who is responsible for the patient's care should be identified. When involving family in such circumstances, it is helpful to pay attention to the apparent needs of the family members and to the communication patterns between the family and the patient. Always explain your expectations so that everyone present understands:

- *(Dentist to mother of fidgety child)* "Many boys and girls get antsy sitting through an appointment like this. Perhaps you could help me by holding Jamie's hands."
- *(Dentist to husband of elderly patient)* "Ruth is going to need your help for the first few hours following these extractions. I'll explain what I expect each of you to do."
- *(Dentist to mother, father, and teenaged orthodontic patient)* "Orthodontic care is a family commitment. Besides the financial obligation, it involves a need to follow the treatment regimen."

CASE: SWEET TOOTH

Gladys is an attractive 13-year-old with a bubbly personality, a gorgeous smile, and an incredibly high caries attack rate. Kim, the hygienist, is shaking her head. She has treated Gladys for about six years and she does not like the changes she is noticing: caries, acne, and weight gain. "You worry me, Gladys. You used to be so conscientious about brushing your teeth and watching what you eat. Now you've got so many cavities. Do you have any idea what might be causing this?"

Gladys just shrugged. Kim continued to stare at her, "Well?" "Who knows," Gladys answered, turning to look toward the windows. "Bad luck, I guess. Maybe its just soft teeth or something." She turned back toward Kim. "Probably you're just imagining them anyway . . . and, so what? A few cavities never hurt anybody."

Kim persisted. "Gladys, it isn't just a few. This visit plus the last one make about eight and that means that something is definitely wrong. Do you want to know what I think?"

The patient turned again toward the windows, "Not particularly. But I suppose you're going to tell me anyway."

"I think you have some problems because of your diet."

Gladys turned around quickly and almost angrily, "My what?"

"Your diet. Why don't you tell me what you eat?"

"Stuff."

"What kind of stuff?"

"Just stuff. Mostly cheeky food, you know."

"No," returned the hygienist, "I don't know. Why don't you give me some very specific examples. What did you have yesterday?"

"Oh, pastry, coke, diet bars, and tomato juice. I don't know. French fried onion rings for lunch and a shake, some diet bars and celery, more onion rings, granola, a TV dinner. I guess that's about it."

Kim moved around in front of her patient. "Gladys, if yesterday is typical, you have definitely got an eating problem."

"What do you know about food," interrupted the teenager. "I read that Brooke Shields eats onion rings and vegetables all the time, and everybody knows that diet bars are good for you."

"Whether you like it or not," continued the hygienist, "the way you're eating is causing problems with your teeth, to say nothing of those blotches on your face and the extra weight you've put on in the last year." Gladys crossed her arms, set her jaw, and faced the windows yet again. Kim proceeded without hesitation. "I'm going to explain to you some basic facts about diet and some ways you can really help yourself. I've also got a little program that will get you eating right in about a month. You don't have to do everything I say because you're old enough to make your own decisions, but you do have to listen to me for the next ten minutes."

ANALYSIS

Gladys has a fairly common teenage problem and exhibits very predictable young adolescent behavior. When asked what she thinks is causing the large number of cavities, she gives *six* different answers, some of them contradictory, all of them inappropriate. Teenagers can easily maintain several conflicting or nonsensical opinions simultaneously, thus making it difficult for adults to reason with them. Gladys' remark that the hygienist is probably just imagining the caries is an example of projection. From time to time, we all fantasize our problems away or project them into the heads of others. Teenagers are very prone to do this and to feel that they are magically protected against evil or destined to success. They have difficulty applying probabilities to themselves.

"Cheeky" food is an example of argot, an "in" word not intended to be understood, but to mark the listener as being an outsider. The inconsistency of using argot in the same sentence with the cliché, "you know" (which implies ability to read the patient's mind), is typical of teenagers. The adolescent's identification with a role model such as Brooke Shields leads the patient to accept her as an authority on everything. A similar example of overgeneralization is the statement that "everybody knows" about diet bars.

The hygienist seems to be well aware of the inconsistent behavior of young teenagers and she responds with appropriate structure. Kim avoids answering the multiple positions Gladys takes. Reasoning, emotions, and justification of her own authority are bypassed in favor of a persistent, specific, structured approach. Her language is plain and to the point, as in the case of "cheeky" foods. The definition is irrelevant; we need to know what the girl is eating.

REFERENCES

1. Erikson, E.H. *Identity and the life cycle.* New York: International University Press, 1959.
2. Bird, B. *Talking with patients* (2nd. ed.). Philadelphia: J. B. Lippincott, 1973.
3. Piaget, J. *Six psychological studies.* New York: Vintage Books, 1968.
4. Piaget, J. *The language and thought of the child.* Cleveland: Meridian Books, 1955.
5. Bruner, J.S., & Goodman, C.C. Value and need as organizing factors in perception. *Journal of Abnormal and Social Psychology*, 1947, 42, 33–44.
6. Hennings, D.G. *Smiles, nods, and pauses: Activities to enrich children's communication skills.* New York: Citation Press, 1974.
7. Chambers, D.W. Communicating with the young dental patient. *Journal of the American Dental Association*, 1976, 93, 793–799.
8. Ginott, H.G. *Between parent and child: New solutions to old problems.* New York: Avon Books, 1965.
9. Chambers, D.W. Managing the anxieties of young dental patients. *Journal of Dentistry for Children*, 1979, 37, 363–374.
10. Piaget, J. *The child's conception of the world.* Totowa, New Jersey: Littlefield, Adams & Company, 1965.

11. Elkind, D. Understanding the young adolescent. *Adolescence*, 1978, 13, 127.
12. Albino, J.E., Tedesco, L.A., & Phipps, G.T. Social and psychological problems of adolescence and their relevance to dental care. *International Dental Journal*, 1982, 32, 184–193.
13. Farb, P. *Word play: What happens when people talk*. New York: Bantam Books, 1974.

EXERCISES

9–1. Practice active listening with a child or older person. Place the verbal content "on hold" and ask questions of yourself such as "why would they be telling *me* this?" "Do their words suit the occasion?" "Are their nonverbals consistent?"

9–2. How would you manage a 75-year-old patient who cries?

9–3. A child patient asks you, "Does everybody get gas in your office (nitrous oxide–oxygen analgesia)?" How would you respond to the child if he or she were (a) 4, (b) 7, or (c) 14?

9–4. The message below is delivered by a dentist to the patient. Write a translation as you think the patient hears it assuming that the patient is (a) a toddler, (b) a preadolescent, or (c) an older person.

> There seems to be a small fracture or crack in the tooth. It may cause some discoloration but I don't think it will affect vitality. I'll have my assistant take some radiographs just in case.

DISCUSSION OF EXERCISES

9–1. Active listening is critical when dealing with others who do not share your point of view. For patients such as those discussed in this chapter, the verbal content is often of little value and the contextual factors carry the true message.

9–2. The crying of an older person is handled just as one would respond to a young child. First try to determine why they are crying. Normal emotional release is managed with patience and empathy. But some older patients cry as a means of manipulation. You may also want to be on the lookout for bottled up feelings that are not being expressed.

9–3. **a.** Preschooler. "What would you do if I gave you gas?" Find out what the child has in mind—he or she may have you confused with a filling station.

b. Young child. "Would you like to have gas?" Find out how the child thinks he or she will respond—there may be a fear of loss of control.

c. Adolescent. "Who told you that?" Find out what they have heard and what expectations they have.

Generally, unusual questions should be answered with a question. A simple "yes" or "no" or an explanation makes the often risky assumption that you understand all that is behind the question.

9–4. **a.** Toddler. Probably understands nothing of what you say. Forms impressions of how you say it, i.e., tone of voice, facial expressions. The parent, if present in this example, will likely be uncertain about several terms such as "discoloration" and "vitality."

b. Preadolescent. "The tooth is broken and may even have a part missing. It will turn black or green or red. X-rays are also going to be taken for some reason."

c. Older patient. "I'm falling apart again. I'm going to have to have something inconvenient done. The doctor is very efficient and insensitive."

10

Interviewing and History Taking

An effective patient interview accomplishes more than gathering accurate medical and dental information. It also provides insight into how patients respond to illness, defines the respective roles and obligations of patient and professional, and creates expectations for what topics can be discussed and how emotions and status are to be handled (Table 10–1).[1,2]

This chapter focuses on systematic, unbiased information gathering that promotes the treatment alliance. In particular, we concentrate on the information exchange that typically takes place at the first meeting with patients. This is where general health and dental data are gathered and where the tone is set for communication throughout subsequent treatment. The chapter introduces the eleven skills of open-ended interviewing and concludes with a discussion of managing patients who are difficult because they are silent, talkative, or seductive.

GENERAL FORMAT OF THE INTERVIEW

There are four stages in the patient interview: the opening, establishing expectations, gathering data, and the closing. These are diagramed in Table 10–2.

The Opening

Because opening remarks are among the most important a dentist or any staff member may make to patients, several should be

TABLE 10–1. OBJECTIVES OF THE HEALTH HISTORY INTERVIEW

Function	Example
Screening general health problems	Identify history of systemic illnesses, allergies, bleeding disorders, and other conditions that affect dental treatment
Determining patient response and attitudes toward illness	Evaluate trustworthiness of patient's dental and general information and importance placed on dental health as clues to type of therapy patient will elect and extent of cooperation
Defining roles of professional and patient	Establish professional responsibilities of dentist and cooperation expected of patient
Establishing communication rules	Develop expectations about how needs are to be expressed and responded to, e.g., degree of formality, trust, taboo subjects, personal revelation

memorized. An effective opener is a general open-ended question that invites patients to explain what *they* think is important. Many patients are only conditionally cooperative until they believe that the professional will respond to their chief complaint. Typical examples of openers that elicit information while simultaneously establishing the professional as qualified and caring include:

- "I would like to hear about your problem. What brought you in today?"
- "How can I help you?"

Contrast these unstructured opening remarks with the overly structured and task-oriented comment:

TABLE 10–2. FOUR STAGES OF THE PATIENT INTERVIEW

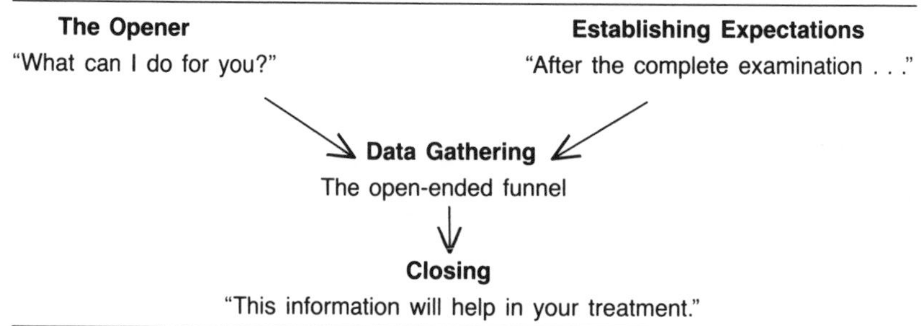

- "Let's see what's wrong here (picking up the mirror and exploring)"
- "Did you complete the health history form?"

Establishing Expectations
In contrast to the "opener," establishing expectations is highly structured. Part of the patients' uneasiness in the dental office stems from not knowing what will happen. On the first visit, it is helpful to explain the sequence of steps, why these are being done, and how long each will take. Again, this is such a typical situation and so important that a standard explanation like the following should be developed.

- "I can imagine how that discoloration on your teeth must bother you (acknowledge chief complaint as important). There are several things we can do for you (promise attention, but not results or satisfaction). I will want to examine your mouth very carefully and take some x-rays to see what is causing that problem and whether there are any other problems (overview of appointment). But first I like to just talk with my patients for a few minutes to get to know them better (announce expectations for treatment alliance). I also want to review this medical history to be certain that there will be no complications in your case (focus on health history).

Information Gathering
The third stage, actually collecting information from the patient, makes use of a group of skills that include questioning, probing, reflection, and others. The information gathering skills are discussed in the next section.

The Closing
The "closing" summarizes key points and reaffirms the treatment alliance. As shown in the example below, the closing should contain an opportunity for the patient to add other comments, a statement of appreciation, and a reminder of the importance of what has happened.

- "Oh, this has been very helpful and I appreciate your candor. Can you think of anything else that you want to tell me?"

If material of a sensitive nature has been given, reassurance of its confidentiality can be added.

OPEN-ENDED FUNNEL INTERVIEW

The open-ended funnel interview begins with unstructured and progresses to highly structured communication. It provides the professional with a general plan for soliciting information from the patient. Special data-gathering skills are required for this interview technique.[3]

Eleven skills can be arranged, as in Table 10–3, from those that allow the patient great latitude in responding (such as facilitation) to those that impose structure (such as "yes/no" questions). Interviewing is the art of judicious selection of those techniques that create confidence and honest answers while generating the needed information in the least time necessary. Taking time with patients initially to listen to what they want to say creates candor and a sense of patient responsibility for his or her own health.[4]

TABLE 10–3. ELEVEN TECHNIQUES IN THE OPEN-ENDED FUNNEL INTERVIEW

Technique	Example
Silence	After asking a question, listen attentively, facing the patient with eyes open.
Facilitation	"I see what you are saying," "um, humm"
Empathy	"You seem worried over the possibility that your teeth are soft."
Summation	"I understand that these pains are coming more frequently and they seem to be at different places each time."
Reflection	"You appear awfully uncomfortable when I mention the bleeding gums."
Probing	"I would like to hear more about why you think 'straight teeth' are important for your future happiness."
Changing topic	"Let's find out what your husband's experience with dentures has been."
Open-ended question	"How do you feel about your bridge now?"
Structured question	"Is it possible that you have ever had heart problems before?"
Reassurance	"Everything is just fine; relax."
Direction or suggestion	"Tell me, is the problem that you're afraid of the expense?"

More structured questions elicit needed information after rapport is established.

Silence Permits Participation

Silence is more than not talking. Silence is a nonverbal technique for showing interest in the patient and encouraging the patient to speak. Saying nothing is an effective part of gathering information. Professionals have to be quiet and listen if they expect patients to tell them anything, and this is a good way to find out what patients believe is important.

Timing is also critical. Silence should be used when it is likely that the patient has more to say.

- *(Patient to dentist)* "My last dentist didn't seem to be all that certain about what to do for this problem." (Appropriate response: silence. This is an incomplete thought and the patient will probably volunteer more information if not interrupted.)
- *(Patient to dentist)* "And that's about everything on the insurance part of the form." (Appropriate response: short silence. Patients should be allowed to switch topics.)

Facilitation Encourages Participation

Nonverbal behavior and short remarks that express the listener's interest are called facilitation, for they encourage patients to continue talking. Head nodding, looking up and opening the eyes wide, or projecting the head forward are typical nonverbal gestures of encouragement. Comments like "I understand," "Go on," or even "Yes . . .," also stimulate conversation. Facilitation indicates that the professional is prepared to learn more about whatever the patient is saying.

Empathy Encourages Discussion of Feelings

Empathy means reflecting back your understanding of another's feelings. Placed early in the interview sequence, this type of response helps build rapport and stimulate more candid, less defensive answers to the questions that follow. Empathic responses show patients that the professional understands and respects their feelings. A patient who seems irritated by the formality and impersonal care received when last hospitalized would likely respond to an empathic comment, "It seems like it bothered you not to know what was happening." This acknowledgment of the importance of the patient's feelings encourages patients to share their reactions to disease and treatment and to provide information useful in planning a general approach to treatment.

Summation Signals Understanding

Short summations that show the professional is listening stimulate further comment without controlling the nature of the response. They can be used whenever the patient has reached a natural pause. For example, the dentist might summarize the patient's comments, "So you've changed dentists several times because you feel they have been prescribing unnecessarily complex and expensive treatments?" It helps reduce patients' defensiveness to hear their thoughts accurately paraphrased.

Reflection Unlocks Suppressed Information or Feelings

We have now reached a point roughly midway in the funnel interview where the professional introduces some, but not excessive, control. Reflection draws attention to an important aspect of feelings or behavior that the patient does not appear to recognize. Patients who are nervous, reticent to talk, excessively talkative, or who appear to avoid or overreact to certain topics can benefit from reflection. By making patients aware that the professional sees the problem, without accusation or judgment, the doorway is open for breaking a logjam of half-hidden feelings and important information. (In the literature, the skill we call reflection is known by the technical but threatening term confrontation.)

- *(Hygienist to patient)* "You don't sound very positive when you describe your diet." (Apparent discrepancy between what is said and the way it is said)
- *(Dentist to patient)* "You seem to be uncomfortable talking about the medications you are taking?" (Apparent discrepancy between topic of conversation and posture)

Probing Searches for Suspected Information or Feelings

Probing directs information gathering to a specific topic and asks patients to give details. The professional may probe for information or for feelings. It is a very useful technique for encouraging patients to discuss their illnesses.

- *(Hygienist to patient)* "So your gums bleed when you brush your teeth. What do you think about that?"
- *(Dentist to patient)* "Tell me about your old dentures."

Because probing exercises more control by professionals, some defensiveness may be encountered. Subtle probing may be nonverbal, such as a puzzled expression, or indirect; "I'm not certain I understand what you mean. . . ." Avoid using the structured and challenging question, "Why?"

Changing Topics Controls Types of Information Available
One more step toward assuming control of the interview is by changing topics. This is a signal that the dental professional has heard enough about a particular subject and directs attention to another matter.

- *(Dentist to patient)* "I see. Now there are some important things I need to find out about your past dental history. . . ."
- *(Receptionist to patient)* "Good. Now can you tell me whether anyone else in the family is covered by dental insurance?"

Open-ended Questions Control Topic but Not Response
Questions that do not force patients to select their answers from a given set of alternatives, such as "yes" or "no", are called open-ended questions. "Tell me a little about your brushing habits" or a general question used as an opening remark are examples.

Open-ended questions allow some freedom in terms of response, but the topic area is controlled and the patient cannot avoid answering. In order to reduce defensiveness, questions must be perceived as an honest attempt to gain required information and not as a challenge to patients' judgment or past behavior. "What have you done about the heart murmur?" has an aggressive quality about it that could cause patients to hide information on that and other questions.

Structured Questions Control Topic and Response
The fastest way to get answers when the dentist or the hygienist already knows what they are expecting is the structured question. "Does this hurt?" "Have you ever had . . .?" "How long ago . . .?" are typical examples.

It is sound policy to precede all potentially sensitive questions with a brief statement of why the information is needed.

- *(Dentist to patient)* "Now I need some information to prevent any undesirable reactions to local anesthetics or pain medication I might use. Are you currently taking any prescription or other drugs as medication?"
- *(Dentist to patient)* "There are several illnesses that require special care in a dental office. I need to know, for example, have you ever had hepatitis?"

There are several problems with structured questions that

must be weighed against their relative speed. Such questions do little to create rapport and reveal little of patients' feelings or their reactions to illness in general. Because many questions such as "Do you brush after every meal" or "You aren't on any medications, are you?" imply socially desirable answers, they are easily biased. Because the professional using structured questions severely limits patient responses, there is little beyond nonverbals that can be used to judge the consistency and truthfulness of the patients' answers. Finally, the professional who uses very structured questions assumes the responsibility for completeness of the line of questioning.

Structured questions are appropriate for filling in missing detail or to confirm important facts if they are used sparingly after rapport has been established and if it is recognized that they may still produce unacceptably vague answers. "When did you notice it?" or "Does it bother you?" may elicit responses such as "a while ago," "not long," "sometimes," and "a little." At this point, the dentist or the hygienist has two options. To obtain specific answers, the professional might probe ("Could you be more specific?") or simply remain silent implying that a more complete answer is expected.

Subjective experience such as pain, satisfaction, and aesthetics are difficult to report. They are best dealt with by concentrating on behavioral manifestations. "Does it hurt enough to interfere with eating or to require medication?"

Nonverbal communication may be a clue to the truthfulness or completeness of patients' responses. Pauses in unexpected places, looking away, and lowering the voice *could* mean that the patient is censoring the response. Again, probing ("I would like to hear more about that") or silence should be used to clarify suspected ambiguous answers. If it is quite likely that the patient is hiding information, reflection is necessary. "Whenever the topic of your previous dental care has come up, you have been very quiet and given vague answers. Do you think that is significant?"

Reassurance Can Diminish Importance of Patients' Concerns

Reassurance is an attempt to restore patient confidence. When warmth and respect are communicated, this can help build rapport and facilitate data gathering. Typically it is the nonverbal component of reassurance that makes it effective. Frequently, however, reassurance has an effect that is the opposite of what was intended. Patients who are told "not to worry" may feel that their concerns are not important or are silly. Reassurance draws attention away from the patient to the dentist. Empathic responses are usually more effective when professionals feel tempted to use reassurance.

- *(Assistant to patient)* "It doesn't matter what your friends think about braces. Just remember 'braces are beautiful.' " (Response is critical of friends and is too abstract) "I can tell you are worried what your friends might think." (Preferred response)
- *(Dentist to patient)* "Don't worry about that. It's normal. We can take care of everything." (Response dismisses concern with no reason given) "You seem concerned. Would you like to discuss it some more?" (Preferred response)

Direction or Suggestion Exerts Maximum Control

The extreme of authority in information gathering occurs when dental professionals give directions or offer suggestions about how patients feel or what they should do. Such an approach is open to the triple problem of defensiveness, bias, and dependency. Any initial time savings are apt to be swept away by patients who resist what the dentist has decided is best or by cancellations, tardiness, or delayed payments. "Well, you look like the kind of person who wants only the best, so I'll tell you what I propose. . . ." may be an effective way to end an interview, but it would be poor practice near the beginning.

The eleven skills are a menu from which appropriate alternatives are selected to suit the needs of the occasion. Experience and sensitivity are required to blend the right combination of techniques for each circumstance. For example, information gathering in conjunction with emergency treatment is shortened and structured to identify allergies, communicable diseases, and compromising medical conditions. Emergency patients are receptive to more open-ended and complete interviewing following treatment. In general, the more complex the treatment and the more it depends on patient participation, the longer the interview will be and the more it will use unstructured techniques. Routine recalls should be an occasion for reviewing the significant features of the health history and a general probing question about patient feelings can be helpful: "How do you feel about your dental health?" History taking is an ongoing process as professionals constantly update their knowledge of patients.

CUSTOMIZING FOR SPECIAL PATIENTS

Information gathering, in conjunction with building a foundation for further care, is most effective when customized to individual patients. Patient mood shifts must be accommodated. Children and older patients require special adjustments. In addition, there are some known typical sex and cultural differences. Men, for example, are less likely to report pain and discomfort than are women.[5] Individuals of lower socioeconomic status describe their illness in more personal, concrete, disorganized, and segmented terms, and are less objective and sensitive to context.[6]

Three types of patients merit special attention here because their unacceptable behavior most often interferes with the health history. The silent patient, the talkative patient, and the patient who makes personal advances can usually be dealt with easily once the nature of the problem has been accurately diagnosed.

The Silent Patient

The uncommunicative patient is seldom recognized as a problem early in treatment. It is typically after they refuse to follow suggestions, vacillate on a treatment plan, or fail to come for appointments that it is discovered that no treatment alliance has been developed. The truthfulness and completeness of health history and insurance information can also be challenged. Patients may be silent because they are impatient to finish, anxious and defensive, or not energetic. The proper technique for managing these patients depends on diagnosing the cause of their silence.

Patients who are *impatient* to get through the procedure quickly, making minimal responses in order to avoid prolonging the interview, will usually answer "Oh, I'm okay" and may add, "Let's go on." It is valuable in such cases to ensure that the patient knows the importance of the questions and how long the interview will take. In contrast, those who are silent out of *anxiety* or *defensiveness* will gladly engage in small talk. They may deny that they are quiet. In such cases, less structure is helpful to establish general rapport and reasons should be given prior to asking for sensitive information. The third type of patient is *tired* or *distracted* by nondental problems. More animation in the professional's voice and movements helps, but the patient's low energy should be regarded as a clue to avoid asking for complex decisions, and important information given to the patient should be stressed or put in writing.

The Talkative Patient

Sometimes the problem is a patient who talks too much. Again, there is not one type of excessively verbal patient or one response—there are five (Table 10–4). Usually it is easy to identify the cause of the talkativeness because the patient is saying so much. Professionals should be cautious not to use facilitation inappropriately because this stimulates talking.

Some people are *obsessive* and feel compelled to answer even the simplest question in excruciating detail. Others just *fail to understand* because they are nervous or because of poor command of spoken English. These two cases are the easiest to handle. A polite interruption, usually in the form of a summary or a change of topic is sufficient. Patients who are *generally anxious* may also talk too much. An empathic response shows that the professional understands and accepts the patient's feelings. If this is insufficient, repeating the expectations for the procedure will help.

The most difficult patients are those who are talking as a strategy for corrupting the normal dentist–patient relationship. Some expect health care professionals also to provide psychiatric help or fill their *insatiable need for empathy*. Others are aggressive or disruptive in order to control the relationship or *undermine the professional's authority*. In both cases, the professional must remind the patient of their role and the standards of the office. Table 10–4 shows how this can be done tactfully. In many cases, reflection will cause some anger, but the sooner this is done, the more easily it can be managed.

The Seductive Patient

When patients or co-workers have exceeded the boundaries of their proper role by making personal advances, they must be reminded of the dental nature of their relationship. No apology should be

TABLE 10–4. FIVE TYPES OF TALKATIVE PATIENTS AND HOW TO HANDLE THEM

Type	Strategy	Example
Obsessiveness	Summarize, change topic	"Good, now let's talk about allergies."
Poor communication skill	Summarize, change topic	"So, there are really no serious problems in this area. . . .?"
Anxiety	Empathy	"You seem to be worried about having anesthesia."
Excessive need for empathy	Direction	"I see, Mr. Priestly, but I'm sure you came to me to have this denture repaired."
Aggression, control	Direction	"Did you know you are talking so much that I can't proceed with your treatment?"

offered and no judgment made. A professional and nonemotional tone is important.

- "Mr. Barlow, I cannot see how this conversation relates to the problem you are having with your gums."
- "Let's concentrate on your dental work, please."

The problem is that most advances are not conspicuous. Because of the risk of rejection, seductive remarks are often combined with innocent messages. "You have very sensitive hands" is a comment that can be addressed either to a professional or to an amour. Such disguised suggestions permit the speaker to save face and test "which channel the listener is tuned to." The proper response is to stress the literal, professional meaning of any ambiguous remark.

It is imperative that dental professionals avoid any conscious or unconscious behavior that might stimulate personal advances from patients. Encouragement might come from such seemingly innocent sources as telling patients some of one's personal troubles. As this is not customary professional behavior, it may be taken as a sign that the normal treatment alliance can be suspended.

CASE: OPEN-ENDED FUNNEL

In the following brief excerpt from a health history, it is shown how the dentist skillfully selects various communication techniques to draw out information quickly but without excessive control. Extensive analysis of complete patient interviews may be found in several texts.[1,4,7]

Dentist: Is there anything you think I ought to know about your heart or blood system? (Change topic)

Patient: No.

Dentist: Can I assume then that you have had no strokes, heart attacks, etc. (Summary)

Patient: No, nothing serious like that.

Dentist: (Looking up quizzically) (Silence) You look like you were going to say something. (Reflection)

Patient: Oh, I wasn't going to say anything. But I guess you might say my blood pressure is a little high.

Dentist: Yes? (Facilitation)

Patient: Yes, it's about 150 over 90, I think. But that's better than it used to be.

Dentist: That's important. I'd like to hear more about what you're doing to control it. (Probing)

Patient: Well, I'm taking two tablets of Aldoril a day.

Dentist: Are you under a doctor's care currently? (Structured question)

Patient: Oh, yes, Dr. Mailman over at the University.

Dentist: Okay, good. So the only problem you are having with your heart is some hypertension, which you are controlling with Aldoril, and you're seeing Dr. Mailman regularly? (Summary)

Patient: Right.

REFERENCES

1. Engel, G.L., & Morgan, W.L., Jr. *Interviewing the patient.* Philadelphia: W.B. Saunders, 1973.
2. Feinstein, A.R. *Clinical judgment.* Baltimore: Williams and Wilkins Company, 1967.
3. Gordon, R.L. *Interviewing: Strategy, techniques and tactics* (3rd ed.). Homewood, Ill.: Dorsey Press, 1980.
4. Enelow, A.J., & Swisher, S.N. *Interviewing and patient care.* New York: Oxford University Press, 1972.
5. Jaco, E.G. (Ed.). *Patient, physicians, and illness.* Glencoe, Ill.: The Free Press, 1958.
6. Schatzman, L., & Strauss, A.L. Social class and modes of communication. *American Journal of Sociology,* 1955, 60, 329–338.
7. Froelich R.E., Bishop F.M., & Dworkin S.F. *Communication in the dental office: A programmed manual for the dental professional.* St. Louis: C.V. Mosby, 1976.

EXERCISES

10–1. Review a copy of the health history form that you use in your office or in school. What portions of the form contribute to each of the four objectives of the initial health history interview? What must be added to meet these goals?

10–2. Assume that you are going to meet a sales representative. Write an "opener," a statement for establishing expectations, and a "closing."

10–3. A hygienist is preparing to scale a patient's teeth and use the cavitron. The hygienist asks the following question, "You don't have a pacemaker, or any infectious diseases do you?" This is a highly structured question. Can you think of others that are closer to the open end of the "funnel" and are likely to elicit the necessary information?

10–4. Phrase an appropriate communication for each of the following situations: (a) a roommate, spouse, or friend appears unusually quiet, (b) a salesman interrupts and talks at great length but without answering your questions, (c) a new acquaintance of the opposite sex suggests a closer relationship in a kidding sort of way.

DISCUSSION OF EXERCISES

10–1. There are few specific questions, such as about allergies and infectious diseases, that must be asked in the health history. What is suggested is that four spaces about 3 by 5 inches be added at the end of the history form. The dentist or hygienist knows that the history is complete when they can write in the boxes: (a) alterations in treatment necessitated by systemic factors or co-therapies such as medications, (b) general approach to patient, such as quotes that reveal patient values or attitudes toward disease and treatment, (c) variations from the typical treatment alliance; examples of specific patient expectations or expressed hope are helpful, and (d) communication is clear and rapport established as shown by quoting patient words, which can later be used in case presentation.

10–2. Opening: "What do you have that you think will help me?" Establishing expectation: "I'll tell you what I'm really interested in. I need some kind of filing cabinet that doesn't make my office look like a library or insurance office. I would really appreciate it if you could show me all you have along these lines." Closing: "That's great. Now that I know what you have I can make a fair comparison. It will probably be a few months before I can decide, but I will call you if I think of any questions." Much wasted time has resulted from not establishing expectations and many unsatisfactory sales stem from want of a good "closing" on the part of the buyer. You can expect that a good salesman will also use a prepared and proven "opener" and "closing." In most cases the buyer will push toward the structured end of the interview funnel whereas the salesman will concentrate on the open, value-revealing end.

10–3. "From the looks of your health history, you're a pretty healthy man. How do you feel now?" (rapport and open-ended). Follow up any patient response with empathy, probing, and summation. "In order to be especially cautious about not spreading infection, I want to check for certain problems." An explanation of the effects of the cavitron should also be given prior to the structured question regarding the pacemaker.

10–4. (a) "Paul, you seem a little quiet today." Do not try to solve the problem until you know what it is and how open the listener is to discussing it. It is not recommended to comment on a child's silence as this will tend to make it more profound. (b) "This makes me uneasy. You're talking so much that I'm not getting the information I need." Reestablish the proper relationship. (c) "Now there's an idea with potential" or some other facilitating remark should help your friend clarify his or her intentions. The offer can be politely declined by answering in a kidding manner that includes an obvious incongruous element, "Sounds great, but I'll have to ask the rest of the staff."

11

Treatment Plan and Informed Consent

The treatment plan is a mutual agreement between patient and professional about what dental work will be done. But it is much more—it covers, either explicitly or tacitly, patient responsibility for regular attendance, compliance with recommendations, and prompt payment. The patient also has expectations about how much pain and discomfort will be involved, what negative side effects might occur, how they will be treated, what the finished product will look like, and how it will function. Informed consent is the legal aspect of the treatment plan presentation.

Treatment plans that do not satisfy both the patients' and the professionals' needs are likely to fall apart even when they are scientifically or technically sound. Not observing the requirements of informed consent leaves the dentist open to possible legal action.

This chapter focuses on the interpersonal dimension of presenting the treatment plan. The first section develops the theme that treatment planning is a partnership. A basic pattern of steps in treatment planning is presented as a model. The second section shows how the pattern must be modified to accommodate anxiety-provoking therapies, dependent patients, and the dentists' own values.

SHARED DECISIONS

Most cases present more than one treatment option. After a thorough discussion of the alternative therapies and treatment sequences, the patient is better prepared to make a choice. With a candid, open exchange, there is a greater chance for patient involvement in the decision and thus compliance with the treatment.[1]

The special knowledge dentists bring to treatment planning includes the alternative therapies available, the fees, complications and inconvenience of each alternative, and the likelihood of each being successful. Essential as this clinical knowledge and judgment are, other factors are also needed to develop the best treatment plan. Patients must appraise the importance to them of each benefit and each possible problem. This is based on their personal and unique set of values, fears, finances, and confidence in the care provider. The interaction of dentists' knowledge and judgment and the patients' values makes treatment planning a partnership of shared decision making.[2] It is as wrong for the dentist to withhold alternatives or prejudice a decision with "Let me tell you what's best here," as it is for patients to challenge the dentist's professional judgment.

The Treatment Planning Dialogue

Table 11–1 presents a basic script for the treatment planning dialogue. This sequence of interactions can be followed for most presentations, telescoped in simple cases and elaborated when the care required is complex or the patient has strong and unusual needs.

TABLE 11–1. BASIC TREATMENT PLANNING DIALOGUE

Steps	Examples
1. Diagnosis	"These radiographs show . . ."
2. Treatment alternatives	"The best approach in such cases . . ., but there are other possibilities. . . ."
3. Benefits, hazards, and patient responsibility	"Let me explain what is involved in each of these choices. . . ."
4. Verify patient understanding	"Do you have any questions about the difference between . . .?"
5. Clarify patient emotions	"How do you feel about these choices?"
6. Discussion	"Is there anything else you need to know to make a decision?"
7. Treatment decision	"Have you reached a decision?"
8. Post-decision encouragement	"I feel pretty good about that, too."
9. Document	(Note on chart)

DIAGNOSIS. The definitive diagnosis is presented as the first step in most treatment planning sessions. Study models, radiographs, and lay language help the patient understand the nature and causes of the condition. Care should be taken to ensure that the problem is not exaggerated.[3] This can cause fantasy denial or create an impression that the dentist is "selling" a padded treatment.

TREATMENT ALTERNATIVES. The patient always has at least two choices—one of which is no treatment at all. In many cases there are alternative therapies or the possibility of further tests and continued observation. It is recommended that the alternatives be presented in the following order: no treatment, the treatment of choice, then each additional alternative in descending order of desirability in the dentist's opinion. Assuming that an economically disadvantaged patient does not want or will not find a way to pay for the best possible care amounts to prejudice. When the more desirable alternatives are presented first, there is a tendency for patients to be dissatisfied with each of the successive possibilities and therefore to elect ideal care. It is a characteristic of human nature that choice increases commitment.[4]

BENEFITS, HAZARDS, AND PATIENT RESPONSIBILITY. Every alternative has some benefits, hazards, and responsibilities that should be described to the patient. In order to make an informed choice, patients need to know the cost, length and nature of treatment, home care requirements, and any plausible negative side effects of the treatment. Some dentists prefer to emphasize the benefits and keep the problems in the background because they regard the problems as details that can be worked out after the proper treatment is selected. Patients do not approach the decision in the same way. Responsibilities introduced after even a tentative decision has been reached will be resisted.

As the benefits, hazards, and responsibilities of each option are being presented in order, patients begin to indicate preferences and rule out some options as unacceptable. Dentists who allow themselves to be guided by patients at this point save time and get firmer patient commitments.

VERIFY PATIENT UNDERSTANDING. As patients narrow their decision to one or two options, it is important to verify that they have an accurate understanding of what they will be asked to accept. It is wise to use the listening technique of paraphrase to confirm that patients know at least the essential features of what they are considering.

- "Now, I'd like to check to see if I've given you a clear picture of what will be involved in orthodontic treatment. Can you tell me in your own words what I have just described?"
- "Could you tell me now what you see as the major differences between the surgery and the alternative of your trying to keep the area clean yourself?"

CLARIFY PATIENT EMOTIONS. After confirming the patients' knowledge of the alternatives, it is useful to determine how they feel about them.

- "How do you feel about these alternatives?"
- "You seem concerned about the cost of the bridge."
- "What do you think about each of these choices?"

Careful attention to nonverbal communication is helpful at this stage in treatment presentation. Hidden values might emerge only in the patients' posture, tone of voice, or in seemingly irrelevant remarks.

Dentists should resist the temptation to change patient values. Apparent changes will be short-lived and may lead to feelings of resentment. The reason for bringing patients' values into the discussion is to make reasonably certain that the treatment selected is one that is supported by realistic emotions and thus one that the patient can see through to completion.

DISCUSSION. An effective treatment presentation may raise many issues. It may be necessary at this point to consider further new alternatives or benefits, hazards, and patient responsibilities. Sometimes clearing away emotional obstructions leads to clearer understanding of the facts.

TREATMENT DECISION. The choice of what work is done in a patient's mouth is always entirely the patient's. This can be acknowledged by inviting the patient to choose a treatment.

- "Now, based on everything we have talked about, what do you believe would be the best treatment?"
- "Have you reached a decision about what you would like me to do, or can I explain anything else?"

- "Don't you agree, we'd better fill that tooth before the decay progresses any further?" (Even the most obvious treatment should not be taken for granted.)

POST-DECISION ENCOURAGEMENT. Treatment presentation is not complete when patients choose and commit themselves to a plan. If there was any uncertainty among alternatives, the patient will have misgivings about the options not chosen.[5] In extreme cases, this anxiety can undo a decision the moment the patient leaves the office.

To protect against this problem and to build good patient rapport, it is necessary to provide encouragement to patients. The positive features of the choice they have just made must be stressed.

- "Good, I think that is a sound choice."
- "Yes, I'm sure you will be pleased with the way this bridge makes your smile look."
- "Fine, this kind of partial is very serviceable. And as you say, we can always evaluate the situation again in the future."

DOCUMENT. The treatment alternatives presented and the patients' decision should be recorded in the patient's chart.

Informed Consent

Informed consent is the legal aspect of treatment presentation. Requirements and interpretations differ from one jurisdiction to another, but three basic requirements at the top of Table 11–2 are generally accepted as the foundation of patients' rights.[6] Some customary qualifiers are also mentioned.

The procedure described in this chapter for presenting treatments involves the dentist helping the patient to make an informed decision. Although this is the preferred approach, it is not required by law. Rather than *choosing*, patients can merely *consent* to a specific treatment offered by the dentist. Because of the potential for abuse inherent in a situation where patients are not qualified to evaluate the wisdom of what professionals suggest, certain safeguards have been built into common law. These include (1) explanation of what is to be done in lay terms, (2) discussion of all reasonable risks, and (3) mention of feasible alternatives.

These three safeguards are known collectively as informed

TABLE 11–2. BASIC CONCEPTS OF INFORMED CONSENT

Standard Requirements
Procedure explained in lay terms
All reasonable risk discussed
Feasible alternative treatments presented
Common Exception
Emergencies or situations where a "reasonable person" would not refuse care
Precautions
Patients cannot waive right to informed consent
Implied consent is not trustworthy
Taking of consent cannot be delegated or transferred
Consent should be documented
Proper consent must be obtained for minors

consent. The reason for explanation in lay terms is to avoid intimidation. Contracts between inherently unequal parties are generally considered void if the superior party gained unfair advantage.[7] A patient may not have to pay for a bridge if the judge can be convinced that technical language was used to coerce the patient into a choice he or she would not normally make.

Risks associated with the treatment recommended by the dentist must also be presented. A patient who suffers parasthesia has an excellent chance in a law suit against a surgeon who failed to inform the patient of this possibility prior to surgery.

Finally, all feasible alternatives must be mentioned. Discussing only one treatment is coercive. Referral may always be regarded as a possible alternative, as is "no treatment."

The basic rule for exceptions to formal informed consent stipulates that consent is not necessary for a situation where "no reasonable person" would refuse care. Medical emergencies usually fall in this category. The problem is, of course, that juries differ in their interpretation of what a "reasonable person" might do. The fact that the patient permitted the dentist to proceed with treatment does not constitute implied consent nor a waiver of patient rights.

No mention is made of dental auxiliaries in this chapter. That is because treatment presentation is the dentist's responsibility, and informed consent is the dentist's legal obligation. It cannot be delegated. Consent to have work performed by one dentist in a group practice might not be accepted as consent for another dentist in that group to complete the work. Informed consent for a minor must be given by a parent or a legal guardian. This presents problems in split homes. The parent bringing the child to the office may not have legal custody of the child.

Informed consent should be documented. In high-risk procedures such as surgery, it may be useful to have the patient sign a document summarizing what has been discussed and stating that it has been understood. For most procedures, a note in the patient's record is sufficient. The documentation should mention the information presented and the patient's response. In some cases, informed consent must be obtained over the telephone. This is often the case for children who suffer facial injuries at school. In such cases, the assistant or receptionist should listen as a witness on an extension telephone and this should be noted in the record.

INFORMED CONSENT VERSUS SHARED DECISION MAKING. Informed consent serves as a defense against suits that are brought by patients against dentists. It does not prevent legal actions, nor does it help to ensure compliance with all aspects of the treatment after it has been accepted by the patient. What is lacking in the informed consent model is appropriate consideration of the patient's values. By contrast, the sequence of procedures in shared decision making builds open communication into the treatment plan at the beginning and maximizes patient commitment to therapy. It also includes the three legal requirements for informed consent.

CUSTOMIZING TREATMENT PRESENTATION

The basic treatment planning dialogue just described must be modified when strong emotions are involved, when the patient attempts to evade responsibility for the choice of treatment, and when the patient and the dentist cannot agree upon an acceptable treatment.

Helping Emotional Patients Make Decisions

When patients cannot cope with emotions generated by some treatment plans, their rational processes are compromised and there is limited commitment and follow-through. When dentists help patients find the resources necessary to manage their own feelings, the subsequent dental experience will be more successful. This requires a small detour in the treatment planning dialogue to assess the patients' awareness of the situation and feelings towards it, and to present the diagnosis realistically.[8]

ASSESSMENT. Bluntly informing a patient of an anxiety-provoking diagnosis such as oral cancer is imprudent and callous. It is helpful to learn what patients already know and what they are prepared to hear in order to pitch the presentation at an appropriate level. The following questions might help.

- "How do you feel right now? How do you feel about your dental health?"
- "What do you know about oral cancer?"
- "What do you understand about the problems you have?"

COPING DIAGNOSIS. When presenting an emotion-evoking diagnosis, a very delicate balance must be achieved between the seriousness of the condition and the possibility of coping with it. It is misleading and unethical not to tell the patient what will happen if periodontal conditions or malocclusions are left untreated. Equally unfortunate consequences result when the patient is made to feel that the damage is formidable and inescapable. Studies indicate that a preparatory message can soften the emotional impact of a subsequent threatening event. To be effective, the message must correctly predict the event, without making the potential danger appear so overwhelming that nothing can be done to avert or minimize it.[3]

- "Yes, periodontal surgery is for some quite uncomfortable. The worst part is over in a matter of days and there are medications, of course."
- "Orthodontic work this involved is bound to be expensive. But there are a variety of alternatives and different sources for money for the treatment."

Threats which overwhelm available coping defenses typically lead to denial. The credibility of the source is denied ("I'll find a dentist who knows what he's talking about"). The severity of the threat is denied ("He's exaggerating for the effect"). One's vulnerability is denied ("That kind of thing only happens to others"). Dentists who present a threat too great for their patients to handle run the risk of driving their patients away.

Patients who are realistically prepared for what to expect under stressful circumstances are better able to cope. In a hospital study, patients who were informed in realistic terms about the normal consequences of surgery and recovery required less analgesia and were discharged earlier than patients who simply were reassured that "everything would be alright."[9]

Once the coping strategy has been completed, the normal treatment planning dialogue is resumed, usually at the point of verifying patients' understanding. The presentation should proceed in small steps, frequently calling for paraphrase to verify understanding and clarifying emotions through empathy.

Do Not Accept Patient's Responsibilities

There are few people in positions of authority who are not flattered by being asked their opinion. In a helping profession such as dentistry, there is a natural impulse to respond quickly to patients' questions and requests. It is tempting to save a few minutes in the treatment presentation and assume responsibility for the patient when invited to do so. "What would you do, Doctor, in this case?" Sometimes with a hostile patient the dentist accepts unrealistic responsibility in reaction to challenges such as, "You're the doctor. I'm paying you to know what has to be done."

HELPING PATIENTS DECIDE. There are two reasons why dentists should accept as little responsibility as possible for determining treatment. Legally, it is a nontransferable right of patients to determine what will be done with and to their body. The second reason why patients must accept responsibility is the commitment this creates. The more patients believe they have succeeded in transferring responsibility to the dentist, the less they are likely to master oral hygiene habits, follow through on postoperative instructions, appreciate the work done, or pay for it.[5] The dentist who has been given all the credit for fixing patients' teeth can expect to receive all the blame when the treatment deteriorates.

The discussion step in treatment planning is often the time when the dentist can detect patients who hesitate to accept responsibility. The appropriate response for the dentist is to probe the basis for the reluctance or, if necessary, draw the patients' attention to the fact that they are not making a decision.

- "Yes, it really is a tough decision. It is always difficult to compare costs and benefits."
- "You seem undecided between the two types of bridge."
- "You seem to be waiting for me to tell you what you should do."

Patients often avoid responsibility because of the tension involved in trying to decide between two very similar alternatives. The dentist can help by clarifying and shedding new light on the alternatives. This involves redirecting the patient back to the step in the treatment planning dialogue where the patients' understanding is verified.

When patients confront dentists with a direct request that the professional assume responsibility for the choice, dentists should respond with an assertive response.

- "I can help you as much as you want with the facts of the choice, but I can't make the decision for you because every individual has his or her own values and preferences."

BE CAUTIOUS IN GIVING ADVICE. There are hidden dangers in responding to patient requests for advice. Sometimes questions are cleverly disguised ploys to delay fearful situations, such as injections. At other times questions might be used to distract the dentist from the customary professional role. Advice on hairstyles or investments reduce the dentist's status. A significant problem in giving advice is the danger that it will be taken out of context.

There are three rules for giving advice. First, find out what the patient already knows or thinks about the area in question. Second, find out why they want the information. Third, find out what they intend to do.

Dentists should be particularly sensitive to questions involving drugs and to questions from mothers about their children's development. Questions about treatment philosophy are often tests to determine whether the dentist can give answers corresponding to the opinions that patients already have. Much confusion and surprise can be avoided by probing the reason for the questions before attempting to answer.

Maintain Your Own Standards

Respect for patients' values in treatment planning does not mean that the dentist has to abandon his or her own. The treatment planning dialogue suggested here works to ensure professional integrity by means of clearly identifying the dentist's and patients' values.

After patients have chosen a treatment that is acceptable to them, three possibilities exist: (1) the patients' choice may be acceptable to the dentist, (2) it may be partially acceptable, but compromised, or (3) it may be unacceptable to the dentist. When the patient wants care that the dentist considers compromised or unacceptable, the treatment planning dialogue must be modified.

HANDLING COMPROMISED TREATMENT. When dentists agree to perform a treatment that is felt to be less than ideal, they should make the patient aware of this fact. An assertive I-message is appropriate. It reminds the patient of the dentist's integrity without engendering a defensive reaction.

- "Okay, I will replace the facing. And I think we can make it very presentable and functional. I would have preferred to replace the entire bridge; it will possibly have to be done soon anyway, as I explained."
- "Yes, I can go ahead with the treatment even without the x-rays. But I have those reservations that I mentioned before. This is important to me so I would like to confirm that you understand the risks."

HANDLING UNACCEPTABLE TREATMENT. Occasionally, a patient will insist on a treatment that is unacceptable to the dentist. A patient may request that sound teeth be extracted or may refuse anesthesia. These situations are also handled with an assertive I-message.

- "I won't try to change the way you think about this. But I hope you can respect me when I repeat that these teeth do not have to be extracted and so you will have to have it done by another dentist."
- "I respect your feelings about privacy and not wanting to have tests you consider to be unnecessary. But I cannot afford the risk to my other patients of treating someone with a possible history of hepatitis, except on an emergency basis. If you wish, I can recommend several other dentists and you can consult with them about care, although I would expect that they might feel the same."

In cases of compromised and unacceptable treatments, the dentist should document the patient's choice and the reasons given by the dentist about possible hazards in the compromised treatment or the reasons for declining treatment. When the patient insists on an unacceptable treatment, the dentist should offer to assist the patient in finding alternative care. When referring patients, it is prudent to offer at least two names, leaving the final choice to the patient. If patients sue the dentist to whom they have been referred, they will likely name the referring dentist as codefendant if it appears that the patient had no choice.

CASE: SHARING THE DECISION

Dentist: (Diagnosis) Mr. Barris, the x-rays confirm that all three of these teeth are pretty badly decayed. This one here is the worst. That is the one you say is causing you some discomfort.

Patient: I see . . .

Dentist: (Treatment alternatives) There are several options. Of course, if nothing were done the decay would progress into the pulp of the teeth. That may be painful and requires either extraction or root canal therapy. This molar may already be so far decayed that it cannot be filled in the usual way. The other two are okay, if we put in silver fillings right away. On the molar we could try a filling with protective material under it or we could go straight for root canal therapy.

Patient: You can save the others, you say. But I don't understand about the molar. That's the one that hurts now, right?

Dentist: (Benefits, hazards, and patient responsibility) Right. Let me explain. The conservative approach is to attempt a large filling. When I get in there, we may find that it won't work. Even if it does, it is likely to cause new problems in a few years. The other approach is to remove the pulp now, do a root canal, and cover it with a crown. I could do all the fillings in one appointment if you elected that treatment. The root canal would take three or four visits and would cost about $650 as compared to $70 for the fillings. (Verify patient understanding) Is it clear what your choices are?

Patient: I think so . . .

Dentist: Maybe you could put it in your own words, Mr. Barris, so I can see if I've made myself clear.

Patient: I'll try: I can either get a big filling now which is likely to go to pot anyway or I can go for the expensive root canal work right now. Right?

Dentist: That's essentially correct. (Clarify patient emotions) How do you feel about that, Mr. Barris?

Patient: Well, I'm not exactly tickled about it. It sounds like either way I lose.

Dentist: (Discussion) I agree that these are not the happiest of choices. Do you have any other questions?

Patient: Yeah. Can you tell how close the decay is to the pulp now and how long the filling will last?

Dentist: (Return to benefits, hazards, and patient responsibility) The decay on the x-rays appears close but not contacting the pulp. As for the filling, I can't give any guarantees on the future of this kind of restoration. I have seen some last as long as five years. But it is also very possible that I won't even be able to place a filling in the first place. (Verify patient understanding) Does this clarify things for you?

Patient: Yes, I know you can't make any promises. But if you started the filling and it looked bad, you could decide then to go to the root canal?

Dentist: That's right. (Pause to invite patient to make treatment decision.)

Patient: I really think I'd like to keep this as simple as possible right now. Why don't we try the filling and then if you can see it's not going to work, let me know, okay?

Dentist: (Post-decision encouragement) Fine. That's a good strategy because it keeps the options open. (Dentist also documents in chart which alternatives were presented and the fact that the patient chose the restoration with a later option to include endodontic therapy.)

REFERENCES

1. Vroom, V.H. & Yetton, P.W. *Leadership and decision making.* Pittsburgh: University of Pittsburgh Press, 1973.
2. Chambers, D.W. A general model for the evaluation of potential research projects in the behavioral sciences in dentistry. *Journal of Dental Research,* 1980, 59, 1307–1321.
3. Chambers, D.W. Coping with stress. In S.S. Boundy & N.I. Reynolds, (Eds.), *Current concepts in dental hygiene* (vol. III.). St Louis: C.V. Mosby, 1979, pp. 155–168.
4. Khandwalla, P.N. *The design of organizations.* New York: Harcourt, Brace & Jovanovich, 1977.
5. Festinger, L. *A theory of cognitive dissonance.* Stanford, Calif.: Stanford University Press, 1957.
6. Zinman, E.J. Questions and answers regarding informed consent. *Journal of the Western Society of Periodontology,* 1976, 24.
7. Anderson, R.A., Kumpf, W.A., & Kendrick, R.E. *Business law: Principles and cases.* Cincinnati: South-Western Publishing Company, 1971.
8. Froelich, R.E., Bishop, F.M., & Dworkin, S.F. *Communication in the dental office: A programmed manual for the dental professional.* St Louis: C.V. Mosby, 1976.
9. Egbert, L., Battit, G., Welch, C., & Bartlett, M. Reduction in postoperative pain by encouragement and instruction of patients. *New England Journal of Medicine,* 1964, 240, 825–827.

EXERCISES

11–1. Think back to your last unsatisfactory experience of having a car serviced or work done on your house. Use Table 11–1 as a guide and list those steps that were omitted. How did it make you feel?

11–2. Think back to a situation where you were surprised when a friend or acquaintance reneged on an understanding you thought had been reached. Again, follow the steps in Table 11–1 and identify those that had been skipped.

11–3. How would you respond to a patient who asks, "What do you think about having your hair analyzed to see if you are deficient in your diet?"

11–4. How would you respond to a patient who says, "I don't really think I understand well enough to make a choice. You just go ahead and do what is best."

DISCUSSION OF EXERCISES

11–1. With the possible exception of diagnosis and decision making, it is likely that all other steps were omitted or given very light treatment. If a single "take it or leave it" alternative were presented, this would work to anger most customers.

11–2. Understandings come apart because circumstances change and because they never should have been made in the first place. Skipping steps in the shared decision process increases the odds of an "apparent" understanding, one that either or both patients cannot really live with and that will erode given even the slightest opportunity.

11–3. "I've read several conflicting accounts. What have you heard." This response accepts the question as legitimate but reflects it back on the patient in an effort to find out what is known and of what use your opinion might be.

11–4. The patient is evading responsibility and denying that informed consent has been given. You might suggest, "I'm going to give you the best treatment I can. But I want to make certain you know what I'm doing so you can maintain your own oral health."

12

Compliance With Professional Suggestions

Many of the things dentists expect of patients take place outside the office. Wearing orthodontic appliances, postsurgical regimens, sound diet practices, payment for services, oral hygiene, and prompt arrival for appointments are some examples. Dental professionals typically experience excellent conformance with suggestions when patients are in the office and disappointing compliance when these same patients leave. Although most of the research on this problem has been done in medicine, the following generalizations are apt to be true of most dental practices: compliance ranges widely with situational factors and characteristics of the patient, suggestions that are easy to accomplish and have dramatic effects are more often followed, initial conformance dissipates rapidly, and professionals are likely to overestimate the extent of compliance and have difficulty accurately predicting which patients will comply.[1,2]

One factor consistently found to contribute substantially to compliance is the interaction between patient and professional. Both the emotional and informational quality of communication are significant.[3] Commonly, half of all patients forget or misunderstand some important part of what they have been told within a week; by contrast, those who feel that their needs have been attended to or who accurately recall what they have been told are most likely to follow the professional's suggestions.

Patient compliance outside the dental office is thus fundamentally a communication problem. The most effective strategy is to help patients develop a sense of responsibility for their behavior. This approach and its consequences is contrasted with the available alternatives. Then, three tactical elements—expectations, opportunity, and proximity—are explained as ways to strengthen the effect of shared responsibility.

SHARED RESPONSIBILITY STRATEGY

Patient cooperation has both a direct or short-term aspect and a long-range, indirect one. Some communication strategies favor compliance while the patient is in the office; others are less efficient in such immediate circumstances but pay off with overall superior cooperation. There is also a third strategy that achieves neither. These communication styles are known respectively by the names "autocratic," "shared responsibility," and "laissez-faire," and they are summarized in Table 12–1.[4]

Autocratic Communication

Autocratic dental professionals assume responsibility for their patients' behavior. They give directions, organize, restrict choices, and rely on their own status and expertise. Since they "know what is best for the patient," the major communication tack is persuading others to see things the way the professional does.

- *(Dentist to patient)* "I have found it works best if all of my patients go through a complete workup and then see the

TABLE 12–1. THREE COMMUNICATION STRATEGIES AND THEIR EFFECTS ON PATIENT COMPLIANCE AND FEELINGS

	Autocratic	Shared Responsibility	Laissez-faire
Example	"I like to have all my patients use this valuable device."	"Would you like to see some of the ways you can care for your new appliance?"	"Any questions . . . ?"
Behavior *in* office	Very high compliance	High compliance	Low compliance
Behavior *out of* office	Low compliance	Moderately high compliance	Low compliance
Interpersonal feelings	Tendency to frustration	Support and respect	Neutral attitude or indifference

hygienist until their oral hygiene is under control, then I will be able to see what needs to be done."

- *(Hygienist to patient)* "We teach the method of flossing which has been found to work best, so I suggest you get started right away."
- *(Receptionist to patient)* "Now our payment policy is always to send statements on the fifteenth of the month."

The advantages of autocratic communication are obvious to a busy practitioner. It saves time, usually secures immediate cooperation, and elevates the professionals' status and sense of control. Additionally, in most cases the dentist and staff really do know what is best.

But more is needed than "being right" when the professional must ultimately rely on patient behavior outside of the controlled environment of the office. The disadvantages of autocratic communication include rapid erosion of initial compliance once the authority figure is no longer present and a tendency toward frustration and apathy. Deciding in advance what is best for all patients fails to take advantage of the individuality of each patient. Because these negative side effects seldom occur in the presence of a controlling dentist, hygienist, or receptionist, the effectiveness of autocratic methods tend to be overrated, and patients with unexplainable, noncooperative behavior are written off as being "unmotivated."

The typical pattern in an autocratic practice is efficient control of patient behavior in the office with more than normal levels of cancellations and late payments, and patients who, uninterested in their oral hygiene, are generally and inexplicably not living up to their end of the bargain.

Shared Responsibility

Professionals who set general guidelines and work with patients to find mutually satisfactory solutions build trust, patient responsibility, and commitment beyond what is immediately expedient.[4,5] When patients realize that they own part of the problem of posttreatment self-care, oral hygiene, and payment for services and when they participate in the solution, their sense of responsibility remains after leaving the office. When they perceive that the professional is helping them solve *their* problems, an additional social motive is supplied.

The three examples of autocratic communication given above could be handled as follows when sharing responsibility.

- *(Dentist to patient)* "In our office, I thoroughly examine all new patients and then present complete information to help make decisions before treatment is done. Because we feel prevention of dental disease is very important, all patients also receive instruction from our hygienist. Does this approach sound acceptable to you?"
- *(Hygienist to patient)* "The important thing is to get that plaque off. Let me show you one way that seems to work for a lot of people."
- *(Receptionist to patient)* "We need some kind of regular payback schedule. Tell me, does this meet your needs if . . .?"

The cost of sharing responsibility with patients is a slight initial decrease in efficiency and some loss of status for the controlling type of professional. To be effective, this strategy requires that professionals recognize that most patients have a need to be involved in all treatment decisions.

The major benefit of this communication strategy is patient compliance almost as high outside of the office as in the presence of authority figures. In contrast to patients who are told what to do, those who decide for themselves to pay in four equal installments, reduce frequency of sugar intake, or fill a prescription for medication will do so more readily. These patients are loyal to the practice and more likely to recommend it to their friends.

Sharing responsibility involves customizing care around patients' needs and values. Dentists or hygienists who present the same oral hygiene program to all patients are satisfying their own needs, not those of the patients. Such mismatching of treatment with needs is bound to increase the incidence of failure regardless of technique used.[6] Patient motives for adopting flossing have been found to be a better predictor of continuation of the habit than the technique used to teach it.[7] Of those patients who start flossing because they value professional advise or follow an authority request, only 15 percent are still following suggested procedures six months later. Of those who start in order to avoid specific problems such as periodontal surgery, 60 percent have quit in half a year. The strongest motive, wanting to maintain a generally prohealth life-style, leads to a continuing of the habit in almost all cases. "Behavior modification" techniques for oral hygiene[8] or diet modification[9] are based on drawing out individual patient needs and guiding patients in small steps to assume increasing responsibility for their behavior.

Laissez-Faire Communication

Laissez-faire is a French term that can be interpreted as "do what you want." Responsibility is avoided in an effort to save time and reduce influence on others in exchange for no interference in one's own life.

Such cultured indifference might be expressed as follows:

- *(Dentist to patient)* (Offer no explanation, but proceed with initial appointment and rescheduling.)
- *(Hygienist to patient)* "Whether you succeed or not is entirely up to you. I have shown you what to do, and now it's not my problem."
- *(Receptionist to patient)* (Say nothing about payment) or "We'll work out something for your payments."

This strategy is not recommended because it leads to poor and unpredictable patient compliance both in the dental office and later. It also has a negative psychological impact, creating an impression of indifference, lack of caring, or discouragement.

THREE TACTICS FOR COMPLIANCE

Expectations, opportunity, and proximity are three tactics that facilitate patient compliance. For example, consider a patient who agrees to be tested for hepatitis before starting dental treatment. Which of the following receptionists is best serving the needs of the patient and practice?

- "Let us know when everything is okay, Mr. Wong." (No tactics)
- "Most patients find it convenient to phone one of these four clinics. You're welcome to use my phone if you like." (Indicated what is expected of "most patients," gives Mr. Wong the "opportunity to use my phone," and takes advantage of the proximity of space and time in the office.)

Using Expectations to Guide Behavior

Expectations are suggested norms, guidelines, or accepted standards of behavior that are part of the treatment alliance. Professionals invariably have expectations for patient medications and oral hygiene among other behaviors, but a frequent problem is *failure to communicate these expectations to patients.* Patients who have to guess what they are supposed to do often do not comply.

Establishing expectations is typically subtle and flexible.

- *(Dentist to patient)* "This is the pain medication that most people find very effective."
- *(Hygienist to patient)* "I think you'll find this is an easier way to hold the floss."
- *(Receptionist to patient)* "If you find it's impossible to make this appointment—like if you're sick—please phone to let us know the day before so someone else can have the time."

These expressions of expectation let the patient know what you want and suggest that you believe the patient is capable of the responsibility. Occasionally, your expectations will create difficulty for the patient and you must be flexible enough to negotiate an understanding that the patient is capable of honoring.

- *(Patient to dentist)* "I really do want that bridge but I'll be honest, I can't afford it . . . even in three monthly installments."
- *(Dentist's response)* "Well, let's see if we can't come up with something that is acceptable to both of us. What can you realistically afford each month?"

Opportunity Precipitates Intentions Into Action

The difference between clear expectations or good intentions and following through on a commitment is usually a matter of opportunity. Something specific and concrete is needed to get things started.

- *(Hygienist to patient)* "When you come back next time I want you to show me how well you've mastered flossing."
- *(Receptionist on phone to patient)* "Hello, Mrs. Kilpatrick. This is Ralph Bradley in Dr. Winger's office and I just wanted to say we're looking forward to seeing you tomorrow at eleven."

There is no effective collection system that does not involve asking for money. Creating suitable expectations helps. Sometimes the opportunity is a monthly mailed statement, sometimes a question at the front desk, "How did you want to pay for this appointment today, Mr. Etzioni?" Some dentists hand patients a written slip at the end of each appointment summarizing the services rendered and giving instructions for reappointment. When the patient hands this to the receptionist, it is a clear opportunity to discuss payment.

Proximity Connects Efforts with Benefits

The closer a commitment is to an opportunity to act, the greater the chances of compliance.[1] Practices that function on a "cash basis," requesting payment at the time of treatment, enjoy a low bad debt level because payment is associated closely with professional service. Overly ambitious treatment plans or dramatic changes in diet or oral hygiene habits invite failure by extending patient responsibility far into the future. Small, incremental plans are more likely to succeed.[9]

Although it is generally impossible to arrange both commitment and compliance while the patient is in the office, it is possible to suggest short-term actions to the patient.

- *(Dentist to patient)* "Do you know where you're going to get this prescription filled?" (Patient must call up a mental picture of filling the prescription.)
- *(Hygienist to patient)* "The first thing I want you to do when you get home is to tape this little calendar on the bathroom mirror. You can use it to record your progress . . ." (Patient begins immediately and has a constant reminder.)
- *(Receptionist to patient)* "Oh, I see your next appointment is the day before Valentine's Day." (Memory is aided by association with a conspicuous event.)

Compliance is a Total Office Responsibility

Oral hygiene, appointments, payments, and many other issues of patient compliance have been delegated by dentists to their staff. Dentists must recognize their high status, which makes patients more likely to comply with their suggestions than with an auxiliary's. Autocratic dentists also may increase immediate patient conformance but make it harder for staff to gain cooperation later. On the positive side, dentists can create clear expectations in patients and make it easier for their staff to encourage patient compliance. Finally, office policy should be understood and consistently applied by all members of the staff. A receptionist who asks for payment and learns from the patient that "the Doctor said last time it was alright if I didn't pay now," has been placed in an awkward position, and so has the practice.

CASE: PRACTICING WHAT YOU PREACH

An ad hoc committee was formed at East Overshoe Dental College to recommend curricular changes necessary to correct the problem that only 35 percent of students and graduates report daily flossing of their own teeth.

Dr. Proforma, Director of Clinics, felt that the problem was even worse. "Not only are the students not under control, many of them give only lip service to oral hygiene instruction for their patients. The two problems are obviously related. How can we expect the students to be effective instructors if they believe so little in prevention that they don't practice it themselves? In my opinion, the problem is in the preclinical courses like Perio where students are not properly motivated."

The head of Periodontics, Dr. Bater, responded defensively. "You really have no proof for that statement. As a matter of fact, our students are exposed to the latest research on bacterial metabolic–host immunologic system interactions. Although we are willing to take the initiative in presenting the scientific basis for plaque control, the problem is certainly more than a periodontal concern. When we ran the experimental gingivitis demonstration on a voluntary basis, only about ten percent participated—and most of those probably cheated. You can lead a horse to water, but there's no clinical follow-through. You grade your students on OHI don't you, Grace?"

Mrs. Curet, Head of the Hygiene Program, nodded. "They also have to get their own plaque under control before they are allowed into the clinic."

"I'm not in favor of that kind of heavy-handed approach," responded the Head of Community Dentistry. Dr. Hopewell continued, "External pressure breeds resentment and compliance only as long as the threat is present. Who knows what these students will do once they graduate. I guess the worst thing would be that they would refuse to treat any patients until they had a Plaque Index of 0.5. The guest lecturer who showed the students how to do plaque control says that Maslow's hierarchy of needs can be used to motivate any patient, and it is all done in a positive fashion."

"Can I say something?" asked Art Major, a senior dental student on the committee. "I think most everyone agrees that plaque control is important and we can certainly *talk* about it after Dr. Bater's course. But there's so much going on in the clinic and so little time in our personal lives that somehow it just gets crowded out. In the clinic you learn pretty quickly what is important and what isn't. None of the instructors say anything about a little plaque in the patient's mouth, but your amalgams had better be polished like a mirror. The big problem is that no one really shows us how to do oral hygiene instruction. Everyone talks about how great and important it is and then they expect you to go down in the clinic and waste your time talking to patients. The one or two students who get turned on to plaque control aren't rewarded enough when faculty are looking for other things. Getting a grade isn't like getting a grade for a perio surgery. I will do surgery after I graduate because I see it works and not because of the grade."

The committee interviewed several more students in both dentistry and hygiene to confirm what Art Major had said. After several meetings, the committee developed the following approach. The Department of Hygiene assumed responsibility for information about plaque. Interdepartmental teams from Hygiene, Community Dentistry, and Restorative Dentistry taught oral hygiene instruction skills to the students. In this way, students gained proficiency in plaque control while faculty modeled instructional approaches that the students could imitate clinically. Students were graded for oral hygiene instruction in the clinic by these same instructors, but students were not held responsible for patients who were poor candidates for plaque control.

ANALYSIS

The faculty at East Overshoe initially made the mistake of assuming that habits would automatically follow from knowledge and attitudes. Research evidence was presented that made sense to the faculty—it may not have been particularly meaningful to the students. Stressing the negative consequences of plaque has limited value as a motivator in the face of so many contrary attitudes that are neither acknowledged nor discussed. No practice with feedback was provided to teach the skills of plaque control or of instruction. The greatest problem was that teaching plaque control was rigged for failure in the clinic.

An educational approach likely to succeed was fashioned only after faculty involved the student "consumer" (shared responsibility) as an alternative to telling the students what to do (autocratic) or giving it up as useless (laissez-faire). Expectations for giving oral hygiene instruction were created by a combination of instruction and grading. The strategic advantage of controlling student clinical activities affords both opportunity and proximity.

REFERENCES

1. Stone, G.C. Patient compliance and the role of the expert. *Journal of Social Issues*, 1979, 35, 34–59.
2. Haynes, R.B. A critical review of the 'determinants' of patient compliance with therapeutic regimens. In D.L. Sackett & R.B. Haynes

(Eds.), *Compliance with therapeutic regimens.* Baltimore: Johns Hopkins University Press, 1976.

3. Hulka, B.S., Cassel, J.C, Kupper, L.L., & Burdette, J.A. Communication, compliance, and concordance between physicians and patients with prescription medications. *American Journal of Public Health,* 1976, 66, 847–853.
4. Lewin, K., & Lippitt, R. An experimental approach to the study of autocracy and democracy: A preliminary note. *Sociometry,* 1938, 1, 292–300.
5. Bonoma, T.V., & Zaltman, G. *Psychology for management.* Boston: Kent Publishing, 1981.
6. Chambers, D.W. Susceptibility to preventive dental treatment. *Journal of Public Health Dentistry,* 1973, 33, 82–90.
7. Boyer, E.M.H. *Compliance with dental regimens: A case study of an innovative dental practice.* Doctoral dissertation, Columbia University, Graduate School of Arts and Sciences, 1980.
8. Weinstein, P., & Getz, T. *Changing human behavior: Strategies for preventive dentistry.* St Louis: C.V. Mosby, 1978.
9. Chambers, D.W. Behavior modification. In P.M. Randolf & C.I. Dennison (Eds.), *Diet, nutrition, and dentistry.* St Louis: C.V. Mosby, 1982.

EXERCISES

12–1. When was the last time you felt like disputing a charge such as for a purchase or a parking ticket? Which communication strategy was used to let you know that you owed something? How were expectations, opportunity, and proximity used? How did you feel?

12–2. Create a payment policy for your office. Identify the places in the history of a patient's attendance in the office where this policy requires communication. Write typical messages.

12–3. Make a list of excuses patients might offer for trying to avoid or delay payment. Next write assertive responses that a receptionist might make in reply.

DISCUSSION OF EXERCISES

12–1. Typically, disputed charges are expressed in an autocratic or laissez-faire manner with a clear opportunity to pay (a bill or even a summons). They lack proximity and are unexpected—people who park in a bus zone do not expect to be detected. Anger and avoidance are customary reactions.

12–2. For example, in an orthodontic office: "A start-up fee of $500 is payable at the initial treatment visit with the balance due on the tenth of each month divided evenly for the next 24 months." An initial expectation of shared responsibility is created, "This is a long-term commitment and we need some way to structure the payments so it doesn't become a burden. . . . Does that sound like something which will fit within your budget? . . . It is better not to send the money with your daughter so we can either give you a packet of 24 preaddressed envelopes or we can send you a statement each month."

12–3. *Excuse:* "I forgot my checkbook."
Response: "Here is a preaddressed envelope. Will you drop it in the mail as soon as you get home?"
Excuse: "I'm a little short this month. Why don't I just make it up when you get this crown finished?"
Response: It would be preferable to keep the treatment and payments in phase. You will be fine with that temporary for awhile. Why don't you mail in the $350 you now owe next month and then I will phone you to set the next appointment?"
Excuse: "Why should I have to pay anything for these dentures? They don't fit any better than the old ones."
Response: "I'm disappointed, Mr. Pyle, that you are trying to get out of our understanding." (Review Chapter 4 for help on assertive responses.)

13

Preventive Instruction

This chapter is about teaching patients preventive hygiene habits such as brushing, flossing, using special aids, or diet modification. Getting patients involved in their own oral care is rewarding. It strengthens commitment to all aspects of dentistry, improves oral health, and extends the longevity of existing restorations.

Teaching prevention is also difficult. It requires expert application of all the communication skills from listening to rapport to persuasion and motivation. Special sensitivity to individual patient's values, moods, and abilities is needed, and thus nonverbal communication is important.

Our discussion of oral hygiene instruction is based on two assumptions. First, communication can be improved by understanding how patients typically acquire oral hygiene habits. Professionals will know better what to listen and watch for, and what to say and demonstrate when they know the forces at play in habit acquisition. The first section in this chapter describes this process and the communication skills appropriate at each point.

Second, communication can be improved by customizing oral hygiene instruction to each patient. Wide variation exists in patients' sensitivity to and capacity for learning oral self-care, and professionals who have the communication skills to accommodate this individuality will experience more success. The chapter closes by considering these issues.

LEARNING ORAL HYGIENE HABITS

Teaching patients to brush or use floss correctly, or modify their sugar intake requires replacing or modifying existing habits with better ones. The professional does not usually start fresh with a student eager to correct a deficiency and needing only to be told and shown what to do. Existing habits, including the habit of neglect, are in place because they "work" for that patient. Teaching strategies that rely on "show and tell," and even those adding motivational pep talks, seldom produce long-term habit changes.

In simplest outline form, poor oral habits are replaced with better ones when the dentist or hygienist points out that the patient's present behavior will likely entail tooth loss, damage to an attractive smile, and higher cost. The professional works with this patient, providing information, demonstrations, and feedback as the patient practices. If the effect of proper brushing and flossing (both positive benefits and negative costs) better meets the patient's values, the oral hygiene skills will become habit. Without a clear perceived need and a recognizable benefit resulting from the new skill, the old oral health patterns will reassert themselves. This is true *despite* the professional's excellent job of explaining, demonstrating, and teaching prevention.

Table 13–1 shows the habit replacement process in schematic form and distinguishes the communication roles of the professional.[1-3] Nothing changes until a person becomes aware that their *existing habits* are failing to serve their *attitudes*. The newly *perceived need* motivates learning *new skills*. The new skill is acquired through *information, practice,* and *feedback*. This skill replaces the old habit to the extent that it produces *results* more in harmony with *existing values*. Effective oral hygiene requires that the professional listen to determine where in this sequence each patient is and then tailor messages suitable to each stage.

Assessment

The health history, initial interview, diagnostic examination, and most conversations with patients provide the kind of information necessary for effective preventive instruction. Four areas should be considered:

1. What is the patient's present level of self-care—brushing technique, frequency, knowledge, dietary habits?
2. What are the dental consequences of these existing

TABLE 13–1. PROCESS BY WHICH HABITS ARE REPLACED

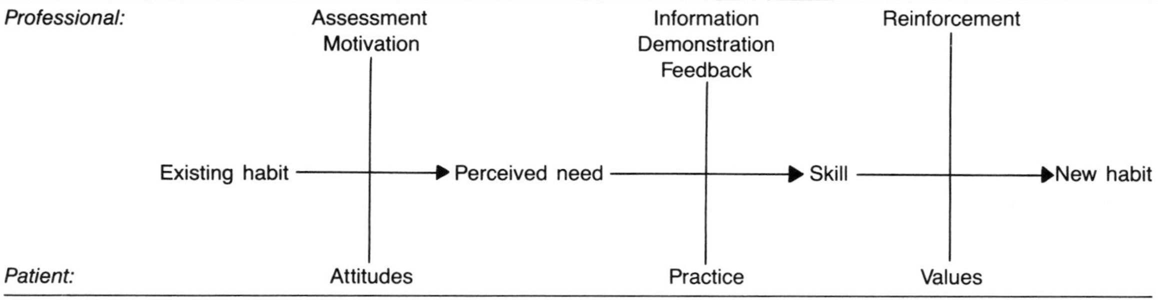

Professional:		Assessment Motivation		Information Demonstration Feedback		Reinforcement
	Existing habit →		Perceived need →		Skill →	New habit
Patient:		Attitudes		Practice		Values

habits—caries incidence, periodontal condition, plaque formation, special restorative needs?

3. What physical factors complicate sound hygiene practices—partially erupted teeth, exposed roots, orthodontic appliances, bridges, lack of motor coordination?
4. What patient or family attitudes or personal or social problems will support or discourage sound prevention—aesthetics, money, personal pride, family disruptions, history of dental neglect?

The preventive assessment is constantly being made as part of normal dental care. Active listening and observation skills are useful. When questioning patients, an open-ended strategy is helpful.

- "Your mouth looks pretty good. Can you tell me what you usually do to clean your teeth?"
- "Since you brush your teeth and floss them sometimes, you obviously know that this is important. Because I want to understand all about your dental situation, I wish you would show me how you brush and floss, in just a few areas."
- "I have just used the disclosing solution on your teeth as part of the periodontal examination. These red areas which you can see in the mirror are plaque. What do you know about plaque?"

Motivation

Patients must be motivated to learn new oral hygiene skills. This is accomplished by making them aware of current habits that are inconsistent with their own attitudes. Patients are stimulated to action when they perceive a need, and this can be most easily communicated when the professional points out undesirable consequences of the patient's behavior. Patients may not always be consciously aware of their needs and attitudes. The professional may have to draw them out.

- "You said your teeth bleed when you brush. I'm sure we can control that inflammation and bleeding with regular, effective flossing. Would you like me to show you the correct technique?"
- "I agree with you; periodontal surgery should be avoided if there is any other alternative, and there is. . . ."
- "You do a fantastic job of regular, thorough brushing and

flossing. It is evident that you are trying. What troubles me is that your caries rate is still pretty high. I'm just guessing that it might have something to do with what you eat. Do you want to talk about your diet?"

Pointing out that the patient is failing to meet the *professional's* standards for self-care may be of little value. Motivation is achieved only when the patient learns that their own goals are not being met. Notice the three-part strategy in each example above: (1) verbalize the need, (2) indicate that it is not now being fully satisfied, and (3) show patients how to do better.

Skill Learning

Patients are skilled when they consistently do what they are supposed to, quickly and with a minimum of wasted effort.[4] Such skill is acquired only by patient practice under the guidance and feedback of an expert. Thus, learning preventive behavior is a cooperative activity to which patients bring motivation and a willingness to perform the task under supervision. The professional's contribution includes (1) planning and arranging the training, (2) providing information and demonstrations, and (3) giving feedback. Table 13–2 presents eleven specific suggestions for teaching preventive dental skills.

Habit Replacement

Habits are self-rewarding skills. The behavior stays in place because it is satisfying to perform it. Patients with a brushing and flossing habit "feel strange" when they skip. Snacking is a hard habit to break because it is intrinsically satisfying. On the other hand, flossing to impress the hygienist, or a child's brushing to avoid parental disapproval are not habits (if the hygienist and parent are no longer present, the behavior stops); however, sound habits may start this way.

When patients have learned to perform a new preventive hygiene skill correctly, one still cannot be confident that it will replace existing habits. The determining factor is whether the *results* of the new skill better serve the patient. If brushing regularly without bleeding is more desirable than brushing infrequently with occasional bleeding, the new skill may stick. If flossing is too awkward, inconvenient, time-consuming, or messy for the perceived changes it produces in gingival health, the patient will gradually lay aside the newly learned skill. Dietary changes are especially difficult to effect because of the strength of

TABLE 13–2. SUGGESTIONS FOR TEACHING ORAL HYGIENE SKILLS

Tactic	Example
1. Describe what is to be learned.	"We're going to focus on brushing and flossing today, and I'll check out your progress next week and then again a month later. I'll also be showing you something next week that you can do for the exposed roots of those molars."
2. Spread training over several periods if it is complex.	"I want to set up several sessions to teach this."
3. Concentrate the supervision at beginning; space it later.	"I'm going to want to work with you about an hour today, then we can just spot check at your six-month checkup."
4. Start with the simplist tasks to ensure early success	"I think brushing is most important and it is something you already do fairly well"
5. Present only essential information and tasks at the beginning.	"The gingiva around your molars are especially inflamed. So let's concentrate on flossing them first."
6. Combine demonstrations and verbal descriptions.	"Angle the brush at 45 degrees like I'm showing you here."
7. Do not cause confusion by introducing too many tasks.	"Okay, I think we will talk about cleaning your partial next week."
8. Reward all approximations of correct performance.	"Good, you've got the circular motion going now . . ."
9. Provide feedback in a supportive fashion.	"Yes, that's right. Move the floss slowly. No, wrap it around the teeth more. There, that's it, good."
10. Review what has been learned prior to adding new tasks.	"Fine. Now let's go over how to position the brush head for the front teeth. . . . Good, you remembered."
11. Continue practicing the entire skill beyond the point where patient first demonstrates competence.	"I know you did a good job last time, but I would like to see you do it once more."

existing habits. Behavior modification techniques, a more extensive version of what has been presented in this chapter, are usually required.[1]

Recidivism (reverting to old habits) is very common in preventive dental education. It usually results from patients lacking supportive values and not from poor professional instruction. In a study of 100 patients who paid to learn plaque control,[5] the reasons given for wanting to learn were very predictive of who continued with the habit. Sixty percent of those who learned hygiene to avoid periodontal surgery or to solve other specific dental problems quit flossing within half a year. Wanting to please the professional or being cooperative were attitudes that only maintained 15 percent of the patients in their new habits. The only effective supporting value was a general positive prohealth orientation that included diet, exercise, and other preventive health practices. *All* patients who saw brushing and flossing as a further extension of this set of values were still practicing their new skills six months later. This was the only self-rewarding value.

There is little the professional can do during the habit replacement stage beyond teaching minor adjustments to fine tune the skill and offering general encouragement. At this point, feedback should call attention to the concrete results of patients' skill and avoid reference to the patient–professional relationship.

- *(Hygienist to patient who has been flossing regularly)* "What beautiful gums! And I'll bet there's no bleeding, soreness, or bad odor now either. I'm sure it doesn't take you long to do it." (Recommended: specific and focused on results).
- *(Hygienist to patient who has been flossing regularly)* "I'm so proud of you. You're one of my best pupils. I wish all my patients could learn to wrap floss around a tooth like you just demonstrated." (Not recommended: too general and focused on professional, patient effort and technique, and not results).

INDIVIDUALIZATION

The objective of preventive hygiene instruction is to create the maximum improvement of which each patient is capable at that time.[6] This goal leads to several strategies for customizing dental health education.

1. There is no "one best way" of teaching oral hygiene, diet habits, orthodontic regimens, and so forth.
2. Patients have capacities for acquiring different levels of oral health behavior. Only a few may be capable of mastering the habits hoped for by professionals.
3. Preventive education is a continual process.
4. Training must be customized to individual patient's attitudes, oral conditions, capacity, and moods.

Readiness

The above section that describes learning preventive behavior as habit replacement is idealized. There are many paths toward the goal—some very circuitous, some with detours, and some that stop short of the destination. Patients travel these paths at their own personal rates—some quickly, some backsliding, some taking long "rests" with no activity. With this image in mind, it is possible to view almost every patient encounter as an opportunity for preventive instruction we can find out whether the patient is receptive.

When people are emotionally and intellectually ready to learn, the instruction is more effective and progresses more rapidly.[7] When they are not, education is a struggle. To determine if an individual is ready, assess the patient's learning ability, oral conditions, and attitudes. Probing statements and other messages introduced in Chapter 10 can be helpful.

Patient readiness typically changes over the course of treatment. The appointment when the diagnosis is discussed and treatment plan presented may not be the maximally "teachable moment." Some patients might be more ready after initial treatment has increased their dental knowledge, sense of pride and investment, and confidence in the staff. Certain patients are more open to instruction directly related to their treatment, e.g., a bridge or orthodontic appliance. After such patients recognize the benefits of what they have been given, they may be ready for general instruction. Other patients might not experience readiness until after a period of "supervised neglect" or backsliding, if at all.

Patients Who Are Not Ready

Some patients refuse preventive instruction or demonstrate by their behavior that they are deriving no benefit from it. For the habit of daily flossing, it is estimated that as many as two of every three Americans are not ready.[8]

These individuals require a special approach in order to prevent professionals from wasting their time and causing a backlash in the patient. When patients verbally or behaviorally express disinterest in learning about prevention, the professional should concentrate on making the patient aware of the effects of his or her existing habits and the alternatives. Teaching focuses on information giving—avoiding both judgment and exhortation. Patients should be carefully monitored. It will be apparent when they want assistance.

- *(Professional to an obviously resistant patient)* "I know, Bob, some people find it difficult to floss, even when they know how effective it is. So if you can find time to do it, great. Let me know when you want help."

There is a danger in forcing instruction on patients before they are ready. In addition to wasting time and creating an impression of insensitivity, ineffective hygiene instruction may actually make it harder to teach sound habits later. When pressured patients build up resistance, they rehearse arguments to support their reluctant position, and rationalize noncooperation.[9] When preventive instruction is subsequently attempted, it must overcome both the initial inertia plus the excuses the patient created to support his or her noncompliance.

Customizing for Children

Preventive instruction for children must be approached in the family context. Children have limited psychomotor skill and limited capacity for understanding the background and rationale of prevention. Although there is considerable variation, most children lack the manual dexterity to brush effectively until age seven or eight and can actually cause physical damage with floss. Children's diets are almost entirely under the control of family members. Therefore, the family must assume responsibility for seeing that children's teeth are cleaned and that they eat properly, as well as for teaching these habits.

The assessment process is more involved when dealing with children. In addition to the special oral conditions and limitations presented by the child, it is necessary to diagnose the family. Who, for example, is responsible for the child's bedtime and eating routines? It might be either the mother or the father, a grandparent, or an older sibling. This person is critical to preventive instruction and should participate if possible. Parental attitudes are influential. There are also domestic circumstances that modify preventive behavior. Ethnic dietary patterns, crowded bathroom schedules in large families, and inconsistent standards for children dividing time between separated parents are example of such factors.

Oral hygiene instruction for children and their helping adults typically takes place in more sessions, involves both adult and child in the skill learning phase, and is more often done in a special area away from chairside. Parents who feel guilty about their children's oral health can be encouraged and indirectly instructed by talking to the child with the intention that the parent will understand.

- *(Professional to five-year-old child, spoken so parent can hear)* "I'm glad your mother brought you in before this got too serious. Now we're going to put some magic paint on your teeth so we can see which teeth need to be brushed the most.

Care must be taken to determine a suitable level of vocabulary for each child. See Chapter 9, "Children and Older Patients," for some hints and cautions. Teenagers can often be motivated through appeal to social convention, aesthetics, or good breath.

CASE: SOME QUESTIONS OF MOTIVATION

Mary Potter, a hygienist, is ready to start an initial prevention appointment for Richard Smythe, a 28-year-old married real estate agent. She has previously reviewed the chart and history for any significant health or personal problems. She introduces herself and converses with Mr. Smythe about his "day at work" and the world economy. An oral prophylaxis is scheduled for this appointment.

Hygienist: Mr. Smythe, before I begin the cleaning, I was wondering how you usually take care of your teeth.

Patient: Well, I generally brush in the morning when I wake up—don't like that "morning-after" taste. Also I brush again before I go to bed. I know I'm supposed to floss, but to be honest, I only occasionally do it.

Hygienist: That's better than many people. I'm particularly glad that you're brushing regularly. Has anyone explained why this is important?

Patient: Yeah, at the last dental office. Also, from all those toothpaste ads on TV. You have to get the plaque off the teeth or you'll get cavities.

Hygienist: Exactly, and not only that, but the bacterial plaque can also lead to periodontal disease and halitosis. Fortunately, as long as we disrupt or eliminate the plaque once a day we can prevent these problems.

Patient: That's interesting. I never realized plaque caused all that.

Hygienist: You're not alone. Most people aren't aware of this information.

Patient: I suppose I should stop eating sweets, too. But that's a tough one—I really love pastries and candy.

Hygienist: I know what you mean. You don't have to eliminate them completely. There are some things you can do to reduce their negative effects. I'll make some suggestions later that may help. Now I'd like to show you what plaque looks like on your teeth. (After disclosing plaque) As you can see in the mirror, the plaque shows up as the stained areas.

Patient: I thought I was brushing better than that. I've got to do better. That performance kinda embarrasses me.

Hygienist: Actually it's very common to miss certain areas in the back of the mouth and behind some teeth. Why don't you brush and I'll show you a few tricks to get at those difficult areas.

ANALYSIS

Presented here is the initial phase of an appointment for a "cleaning." The office in which Mary Potter works does not have a formal prevention program for patients and primarily relies on the hygienist to provide this aspect of care.

Mary Potter has communicated effectively in the assessment and awareness phases of preventive instruction. She reviewed the patient's history to learn about Mr. Smythe. She knows that it is important to be aware of the patient's past medical and dental history, presence of special problems, and personal facts. Knowledge of the patient aids in nontechnical conversation, setting realistic expectations, and enhancing prevention. Mary uses "small talk" to relax the patient and establish rapport.

Mary's strategy is to assess Mr. Smythe's knowledge of dental disease and his oral habits. She accomplishes this with nonthreatening indirect ("I was wondering how . . .?") and direct ("Has anyone ever explained . . .?") questions. She reinforces correct information and habits ("That's good") and deflates Mr. Smythe's guilt feelings ("You're not alone" and "Actually, its very common to miss . . .").

Mary Potter discovered what her patient knows and then supplemented this knowledge. She avoided overwhelming her patient with an abundance of facts, and deferred some discussion until later. Her language was direct, simple, and at an appropriate level without complicated technical terminology.

Mary respects Mr. Smythe's needs and personal eating habits and plans only suggestions for selected diet changes. By avoiding unreasonable demands, there is a better chance for success. Her responsibility is to educate the patient within the limits of the patient's attitudes and priorities. Perhaps Mary will appeal to the patient's need to be free of pain or to his pride.

At the end of the case, Mary Potter commences toothbrushing instruction, and will take into consideration other basic principles in teaching manual skills: evaluation of current manual ability, providing explanations with demonstrations, adjusting to patient skills and avoiding frustration, reinforcement of desired behavior, and using nonjudgmental feedback. (Additional cases involving preventive instruction can be found in Chapters 9 and 12.)

REFERENCES

1. Chambers, D.W. Behavior modification. In P.M. Randolf & C.I. Dennison (Eds.), *Diet, nutrition, and dentistry*. St. Louis: C.V. Mosby, 1982.
2. Lewin, K. *A dynamic theory of personality*. New York: McGraw-Hill, 1935.
3. Whetten, D.A., & Cameron, K.S. *Developing management skills*. Glenview, Ill.: Scott, Foresman and Company, 1984.
4. Cronbach, L.J. *Educational psychology* (2nd ed.). New York: Harcourt, Brace & World, 1963.
5. Boyer, E.M.H. *Compliance with dental regimens: A case study of an innovative dental practice*. Doctoral dissertation, Columbia University, Graduate School of Arts and Sciences, 1980.
6. Chambers, D.W. Patient susceptibility limits to the effectiveness of preventive oral health education. *Journal of the American Dental Association*, 1977, 95, 1159–1163.
7. Ausubel, D.P., & Robinson, F.G. *School learning: An introduction to educational psychology*. New York: Holt, Rinehart and Winston, 1969.
8. Chambers, D.W. Susceptibility to preventive dental treatment. *Journal of Public Health Dentistry*, 1973, 33, 82–90.
9. Festinger, L. *A theory of cognitive dissonance*. Stanford, Calif.: Stanford University Press, 1957.

EXERCISES

13–1. In the following example assess the patient and his dental needs, make him aware of prevention, and plan a strategy for instruction.

> Clark Bingham is a 21-year-old local college student. He is having a very large filling done today and there are several other incipient lesions in his mouth. He brushes irregularly with a scrubbing, back-and-forth motion. He came to the dentist because of pain and was not happy about having a separate appointment with the hygienist. "They just try to embarrass you about how badly you brush," he remarked. "And why should I worry? Look at this beautiful smile; and there's always mouthwash."

13–2. Make a list of the attitudes that support your personal oral hygiene habits. What would bother you if you stopped what you are currently doing to keep your mouth healthy?

13–3. If you are providing care and in a position to make these observations, try to classify patient motives for wanting to learn prevention. How many fall into each category and how successful are they?

- **a.** Prohealth life-style: consistent general pattern of preventive health behaviors
- **b.** Avoiding specific dental problems, such as surgery
- **c.** Trusting relationship with professional and desire to do what is recommended
- **d.** Going along with whatever is required because of social convention
- **e.** No supporting attitudes; not ready

13–4. What is your reaction when you are reminded that you should eat two servings of vegetables each day, eliminate salt, exercise strenuously twice a week, follow all preventive maintenance on your car, and use only the highest octane gasoline available?

DISCUSSION OF EXERCISES

13–1. *Assessment:*

a. Present level of care: brushing only, inadequate frequency and poor technique

b. Dental consequences: reasonably high caries rate

c. Physical limitations: none revealed

d. Attitudes: concern over appearance and approval works negatively (professionals are "fault finders") and positively (sound habits could preserve an attractive smile)

Awareness:

"That beautiful smile will gradually disappear as your teeth continue to decay and as the plaque left by your current brushing habits begins to affect your gums."

Strategy:

This patient must be handled delicately. He must decide that he wants to learn better habits and must ask to be shown how. Pressing him or telling him what to do will likely backfire.

13–2. Share this list with a colleague to see how much diversity is possible. Speculate whether this list is in any way typical of "the average patient" and whether such patients will maintain sound habits without such attitudes.

13–3. No data have been published showing the distribution of patients in these categories. It is guessed that prohealth life-style is not common. If you continue this categorization for some time you will develop a good set of diagnostic questions.

13–4. Of course, we "should" do all of this, and much more. But often it just is not worth it. Many patients regard oral hygiene recommendations as impractical "shoulds."

14

Office Environment and Written Communication

Office design and written material create a mood and a context in which interpersonal verbal communication takes place. Consider how in older banks, high ceilings, marble counters, barred tellers' cages, large checks with formal design, and confusing legal documents have given way to carpeted floors, comfortable furniture, plants, personalized checks, and monthly newsletters. This shift from an image of strength and stability to one of personalized attention to customers has been paralleled throughout the health care profession.

This chapter shows how the appearance of the reception area, operatory, and the dentist's private office project the dentist's personality and create expectations in patients. The latter half of the chapter explores the way forms, records, instructions, educational materials, and signs communicate more than information.

The office environment and written material are *nonpersonal*, as distinguished from the interpersonal communication that has been emphasized to this point. In addition to stimulating general impressions and creating images, nonpersonal office messages differ from verbal communication in the following ways: They are (1) one-way, with minimal feedback, (2) not individualized but common to all patients, (3) used to express status and information rather than emotions, (4) prearranged and always available rather than initiated by patients, and (5) sources of excellent insight into the personality, assumptions, and expectations of the dentist. Professionals who are sensitive to the power and limitations of nonpersonal communication can create an environment to influence patient attitudes.

THE OFFICE REFLECTS THE DENTIST

Furniture and equipment, decor, cleanliness of the office, and dress of the staff are all extensions of the dentist's personality. They are largely subconscious statements of what the dentist thinks the world should be like. An office can express efficiency, formality, control, warmth, carelessness, confusion, defensiveness, or many other attitudes that are quickly read by patients and translated into expectations before the dentist is seen.

Reception Areas Affect Initial Mood

The room first entered should show patients that they are expected and welcome and not add to their anxiety. A casual, informal, comfortable office is signaled by soft chairs and couches, area rugs, magazines suited to the tastes of typical patients, and perhaps some dental health posters. A more formal, professional and business-like atmosphere can be created by formal chairs, wall-to-wall carpeting, green plants instead of flowers, and small signs in picture frames.[1]

Attractive surroundings contribute to a relaxed, confident mood and a sense of energy.[2] High or low temperatures and high humidity tend to reduce communication or give it a negative and critical tone. "Empty" rooms without natural divisions afforded by tasteful arrangements of furniture, as one typically encounters in clinics, suppress talking. The colors shown in Table 14–1 are associated with various moods.[3]

Anxiety in the reception area is heightened by lack of interpersonal contact. There are a surprising number of offices in which no human face is in sight and all that greets the new patient is a closed, semi-transparent sliding glass window and a

TABLE 14–1. COMMON ASSOCIATIONS BETWEEN COLOR AND MOOD

Color	Mood
Red	Exciting, stimulating, alertness
Blue	Secure, calm, tender, soothing, peaceful
Purple	Dignified, stately, important
Yellow	Cheerful, jovial, happy, light
Black	Powerful, strong, masterful

note saying "please knock." In other offices all that is visible of the receptionist is a head showing through a small opening. While it is necessary to separate the patient waiting area from the records and from desk activity, this should be done in such a manner that the maximum human contact is preserved. Closed doors and windows communicate lack of interest, fear of interaction, and perhaps that something unpleasant is being hidden.

Light reading material should also be available wherever patients might have to wait, including the operatory. Magazines with pictures and very short articles are preferable because anxious patients find it difficult to concentrate on reading. Dental publications present the profession in a favorable light and they may be placed in the reception area provided that they contain no anxiety-provoking pictures such as periodontal or oral surgery. Dentists with a significant number of patients who speak a language other than English should subscribe to magazines in these languages and should have written office material translated.

Treatment Areas Reflect Professionalism

Research has shown that modern and aesthetic operatories tend to be associated with patient expectations of trust, skill, and competence of the practitioners.[4] The style of the treatment areas also interacts with the professional's communication style. Dentists with "state of the art" equipment and who also express empathy are perceived as being sensitive. When evaluative remarks are made by dentists with such equipment, they are regarded as "very insensitive and impersonal." The strongest expectation created by modern equipment is that the fees will be high. The operatory itself creates some impressions, as well as influences the dentist's communication style and affects patient expectations.

Laboratories, work benches, and supply closets should probably not be seen by patients, particularly if their disorganized condition might imply that the care rendered in the office is equally sloppy.

The Dentist's Office Permits Concentration

Extended and personal conversations with patients are usually more effective in the environment of the dentist's office. This includes discussion of complex diagnoses and treatment plans, problematic payment schedules, or medical complications. While in the operatory, patients may feel dominated by virtue of their reclining and vulnerable position and threatened by the presence of dental instruments. These circumstances may lead to superficial compliance and shallow understanding on the part of patients whose primary concern is escape from the unpleasant surroundings.

A comfortable environment leads to more accurate recall of facts and more effective problem solving.[2] The furnishings of the dentist's office, which almost always include books, diplomas, and charts, reflect professional expertise that encourages trust. Patients in a physician's office were found to be influenced by the location of the desk.[5] When the desk separated the patient and physician only 10 percent of the patients were rated as being "at ease." When the desk was not used as a status barrier, the percentage at ease rose to 55 percent.

WRITTEN COMMUNICATION

Written communication has the advantage of operating when dental professionals are not present. Forms and material for patients to complete or read, e.g., informed consent or health histories, and mailed material are not always effective communication. Typically such nonpersonal messages are one-way, with no opportunity to verify how well they are understood or even that they have been read. Making matters worse, emotions in written communication are usually minimized and valuable nonverbal information is absent.

Patient Forms

It is common practice for new patients to complete forms while waiting for their first appointment. Typically this includes address and home and work telephones numbers, legal responsibility for minors, source of referral, intended means of payment, and insurance information. A preliminary health history is also usually completed. The effectiveness of such forms is influenced by the clarity of the directions for completing them, how they are introduced, and what is done with them.

The clarity of a form can be improved in several ways.[6] Each required response should be numbered and should begin at the left-hand margin in order to reduce omissions. Series of items such as "Have you ever had hepatitis?" should be arranged so that positive responses are arranged under each other in the same column for quick scanning. Critical questions concerning conditions such as hypertension and diabetes should allow for three alternatives: "yes," "*uncertain*," and "no" to give a greater margin of security to the staff. Questions about patients' age (except to establish legal age), race, treatment for mental conditions, assets, and so on are not permissable on such forms. The rule is that only items directly related to rendering dental care may be asked. Forms should be pretested prior to being produced in large quantities and translated into the languages commonly used by clients of the practice.

Equally important is the manner in which the form is presented to the patient and the use that is made of it. The receptionist should explain the reasons for completeness and accuracy and should offer to help, if necessary. The completed form should be reviewed immediately by the receptionist. Omissions and vague answers can be corrected. A thorough job deserves an expression of appreciation from the receptionist. The patient should be given an opportunity to explain verbally or elaborate on the forms when they see the dentist or hygienist, and questionable items should be explored. Dentists and hygienists should verbally confirm responses on information and health history questionnaires.

Records

The patient chart contains the information necessary for proper dental treatment and is a legal document. It can also be a notebook to aid interpersonal communication. A ruled, blank sheet of paper as the first page in the record, perhaps with a photo, can be used to record comments such as the following: "Grandson to graduate Annapolis June 1987" "Criticized my not *washing hands*" "Doesn't like taste of topical fluoride" "Many questions about loss of tissue in perio surgery." The operator sees these remarks immediately and they will help establish rapport quickly. This type of comment will save embarrassment and give the correct impression that there is good communication within the office.

Patient records can be a source of anxiety for some individuals. Records should not be treated as professional mysteries, hastily whisked out of sight, arousing anxiety and curiosity. Nor should patients be given copies of their charts or radiographs. Such requests are handled by saying, "The usual procedure is for us to mail them to another dentist once we receive a request." Because patients can sue for their records in most jurisdictions, it is important that personal information be limited to factual observations rather than general interpretations—"talks fast and avoids discussing surgery" rather than "scared," or "reacts to local anesthesia" rather than "combative."

Information Management

A variety of information is now mailed to patients. Letters are sometimes sent to patients prior to the first visit thanking them for making the appointment, confirming the time, stating office policy, and methods of payment. Postcard reminders of appointments, particularly for recall, are common. Other types of letters that could be sent include a thank-you letter following initial visit, thank-you's for referrals, a letter acknowledging receipt of final payment after an extensive treatment, or a note of encouragement for a patient embarking on preventive oral hygiene. Some dentists publish newsletters or send birthday cards to child patients. Telephone calls both to and from patients can also be numerous.

It is advisable to maintain a log system for recording all written and telephone communication with patients. This can be done directly on the chart or on a mimeographed form attached to the patient's chart showing the date and nature of any correspondence, billing, or telephone conversation. This will avoid embarrassing duplications and serve as a quick check as to when patients last heard from the office.

Educational Material

Important specific procedures and policies in each office can be communicated to patients in written form. All of this material will be most effective if it can be kept brief, simple, positive, and highly visual. Unfortunately, patients often read these materials while anxious, with short attention spans, and in search of solutions.

Pre- and postsurgical instructions, diet recommendations, philosophy of practice (including total medical evaluation, conservation of teeth, and prevention), payment procedures, recall and routine examination procedures can all be presented in simple outline form. Some of these, such as pre- and postsurgical instructions or care of appliances, should be mimeographed and given to individual patients as appropriate. Others, such as philosophy of practice, should be bound in a binder for patients to read while in the office. Patients who must wait for treatment may be given such material to read. This will reduce the impression of being neglected, and an informed patient can carry on a more intelligent conversation.

Signs

A limited number of signs may appear in offices provided that they contain few words and make a tasteful impression. Logos of bank cards accepted, statement of hours or payment policy, professional emblems, or educational posters in treatment areas are examples. Because patients feel awkward "reading walls," signs should be thought of as pictures requiring only a moment's attention to convey a general impression. A framed typewritten note on office stationary is preferable to handwritten messages taped to the counter.

- "For the health of all, please refrain from smoking in this office."
- "Parents are requested to remain in the reception room until invited to join their child."

CASE: A WELCOME LETTER

On behalf of my entire staff and myself, welcome to our family of patients. Thank you for selecting us for your dental care. We pride ourselves on trying to make dentistry a pleasant experience.

Our primary goal is to keep your oral tissues and natural teeth healthy. In order to succeed, we need your cooperation. This is why we will keep you informed at all times.

During your first visit a thorough examination will be completed. This will include x-rays or other aids that may be necessary to make an accurate diagnosis of your condition. We will discuss the findings and recommend one or more treatment plans, keeping in mind your comfort, appearance, and economic concerns. Estimated fees will be presented and methods of payment selected at this visit.

If treatment is indicated, we will try to restore optimum dental health in as few well-planned appointments as necessary. We appreciate the value of your time and we know the importance of a controlled budget. We expect from you equal consideration in keeping appointments on time and meeting the financial arrangements agreed upon.

We look forward to a relaxed and pleasant visit with you on ________________________. Thank you again for selecting us for your dental needs.

ANALYSIS

This letter creates an overall impression that the patient is welcome and appreciated. It establishes expectations for the first few visits and proposes a treatment alliance that includes sharing of necessary information, shared responsibility for decisions, patient participation in prevention, and adherence to attendance and payment agreements.

REFERENCES

1. Froelich, R.E., Bishop, F.M., & Dworkin, S.F. *Communication in the dental office: A programmed manual for the dental professional.* St Louis: C.V. Mosby, 1976.
2. Maslow, A.H., & Mintz, N.L. Effects of aesthetic surroundings: I. Initial effects of aesthetic conditions upon perceiving 'energy' and 'well-being' in faces. *Journal of Psychology*, 1956, 41, 247–254.
3. Wexner, L.B. The degree to which colors (hues) are associated with mood-tones. *Journal of Applied Psychology*, 1954, 38, 432–435.
4. Jackson, E. Patients' perceptions of dentistry. In *Advances in behavioral research in dentistry*. Seattle, Wash.: Department of Community Dentistry, School of Dentistry, 1978, pp. 17–38.
5. White, A.G. The patient sits down: A clinical note. *Psychosomatic Medicine*, 1953, 15, 256–257.
6. Enelow, A.J., & Swisher, S.N. *Interviewing and patient care.* New York: Oxford University Press, 1972.

EXERCISES

14–1. Think back to your first visit to your dental, dental hygiene, or dental assisting school. What expectations did you develop based on the physical appearance of what you saw? Were your expectations subsequently confirmed?

14–2. Look around the room you are now in. List those things the room seems to assume about those who use it. What does it reveal about the person responsible for arranging it?

14–3. Review and modify an available set of forms used for patient enrollment and health history.

14–4. In any available patient chart, make those modifications necessary for managing interpersonal verbal communication.

DISCUSSION OF EXERCISES

14–1. Common impressions might include status of person you contacted, single or multiple purposes and implications for resources and organization, neatness and cleanliness, how welcome you were. Some students select the school they attend in part on the impressions they receive in these circumstances.

14–2. Winston Churchill is supposed to have said, “First we shape our environment, then our environment shapes us.”

14–3. Numbered responses beginning at left-hand margin. Positive responses aligned under each other. “Uncertain” response option for critical questions. Is there a written explanation of why the form is so important, or is this expressed verbally?

14–4. A place for personal comments and notes. List of all forms mailed by the office with space for date mailed and initials. Telephone log.

Part III

WORK ALLIANCE

The *work alliance* is the unwritten understanding about how everyone in the office is supposed to act. This alliance is the key to a successful, smoothly functioning practice and is dependent on mutual expectation and open communication. Each staff member must understand individual and office responsibilities and priorities and be prepared to contribute and listen to office communication.

The skills presented in the first section of this book are the foundation for communication among co-workers, and many of the issues in the work alliance have a parallel in the preceding discussion of the treatment alliance between professionals and patients. There are five special communication situations involving staff: Chapter 15 discusses the verbal and nonverbal means used to adjust behavior to keep a practice operating smoothly by means of feedback. Chapter 16, "Intraoffice Communication," explores the role of communication in creating group cohesion and participation in the direction of a practice. The next chapter takes up the special skills of "Using the Telephone Effectively." The "Employment Interview" is considered simultaneously from the point of view of the employer and employee in Chapter 18. The final chapter, "Speaking in Public," is the only discussion in this book of verbal, but noninterpersonal, communication. Although the telephone and public speaking may be used to reach patients, they are included in this section because they are also a primary way of contacting professional colleagues.

BENEFITS

Using communication to create sound work alliances will enhance job satisfaction, save time, and promote better patient care. In addition, realistic, mutual expectations communicated among co-workers typically produce two further benefits: improved staff morale and staff productivity.

Staff Morale

One of the marks of being a professional is working collaboratively, guided by common standards of excellence.[1] When the whole staff becomes involved in professional delivery of care, the results include loyalty, satisfaction, personal growth, and support of other team members.[2] A single employee, even the dentist, can be very disruptive to morale if it is felt that he or she is working by a personal set of rules. The attitudes of co-workers affect everyone in an office and are often readily apparent to patients.

Staff Productivity

Employees are more productive when they know what they are supposed to do, when the work is meaningful, and when they feel that someone cares how well they perform their jobs.[3] A rule of thumb in industry is that turnover costs one-half an employee's annual salary.[4] Considering the simple economic costs of productivity lost while a replacement is found, interviewing costs, and substandard performance during training of new personnel, replacing an auxiliary is certainly an expensive proposition.

The costs of retaining dissatisfied employees, including the dentist, can be even greater. Large amounts of energy can be consumed isolating a grumpy or malcontent co-worker or in raising necessary defenses. Patients are also sensitive to offices where teamwork and cooperation are not present.

SPECIAL ISSUES IN CUSTOMIZING THE WORK ALLIANCE

As was the case in the relationship between professionals and patients, there is a common core of mutual and reciprocal expectations at the center of the work alliance. This is displayed in Table III–1. Surrounding these universal needs are rings of increasing variation and individuality corresponding to cultural, personal, and situational differences. It is through communication that we learn about these differences and negotiate satisfactory accommodations or agree to separate amicably.[5]

The fundamental verbal and nonverbal communication skills, such as active listening, empathy, assertiveness, and persuasion, are used to negotiate sound relations among co-workers. But there are two ways in which the treatment and the work alliances differ.

The temporary nature of patient visits makes it easier to postpone solutions or live with compromises. By contrast, the constant and confining nature of the dental office environment requires quicker action and working through of problems with co-workers. Answers that are consistent with the true temper, personality, and talents of the dentist and staff must be found. At the same time that more honest work alliances are needed, it is often more difficult to recognize disruptions. In a busy practice where relationships become routinized, if not semiconsciously automatic, and where communication and attention are focused on the patient, it is often easy to miss interpersonal problems, let alone find the time to address them.

The second difference between the treatment and work alliances is the secondary and supporting nature of the work alliance. The patient is a "silent" but influential partner in any understanding that the dentist and staff reach concerning how the practice will function. Decisions primarily focus on the needs of the patient, not the staff. For example, an informal relationship may be most comfortable for staff members, but if objectionable to pa-

TABLE III–1. CORE EXPECTATIONS IN THE WORK ALLIANCE

Expected of Employees	Expected of All Co-workers	Expected of Employers
Working by a specific job description Loyalty to the practice	Freedom from interference in personal life Personal problems left at home Timely and clear notice of changes which affect others Cooperation and mutual assistance	Monetary compensation Other (fringe) benefits

tients, it is unacceptable. As a general rule, there should be no "personal" problems or "interpersonal" staff problems in a dental office that affect patient care.

REFERENCES

1. American Dental Association. *ADA principles of ethics and code of professional conduct.* Chicago: American Dental Association, undated.
2. Morton, J.C., Clark, J., Adelson, R., & Hornsby, J.L. *Dental teamwork strategies: Interpersonal and organizational approaches.* St Louis: C.V. Mosby, 1980.
3. Hackman, J.R., & Oldham, G.R. *Work redesign.* Reading, Mass.: Addison-Wesley, 1980.
4. Hampton, D.R., Summer, C.E., & Webber, R.A. *Organizational behavior and the practice of management.* Glencoe, Ill.: Scott, Foresman and Company, 1982.
5. Wiles, C.B., & Ryan, W.J. *Communication for dental auxiliaries.* Reston, Va.: Reston, 1982.

15

Feedback

Continuous communication is needed to accommodate the unique pressures of dental practice. The pace, intensity, and demands for consistent high standards of professional care reduce the latitude for personal freedom that employees enjoy in other lines of work. The presence of patients additionally places the staff "on stage," requiring precision teamwork and control of emotions. Dentists and staff particularly depend on each other at chairside. Because dental practice is so complex and demanding it is unlikely that staff relations will simply take care of themselves if everyone is told once what to do. Feedback is the communication skill that permits the constant minor adjustments required to preserve harmony and efficiency in the sensitive dental environment. Good feedback corrects small problems, preventing confrontations, and builds individual self-esteem and a sense of team pride.

Feedback is information from another person indicating whether our behavior is having the desired effect.[1,2] It is helpful to know when we are offending someone or talking too long, whether a co-worker understands what we have said or likes the way we rearranged things. Sometimes we receive verbal feedback when someone tells us how we are coming across. Sometimes we read it in the nonverbal aspects of a puzzled look, an unenthusiastic response, or no response at all. Regardless of the source or whether expressed positively or negatively, the objective of feedback in dentistry remains the same—to draw attention to the consequences of each person's behavior with a view toward improving office efficiency and harmony.

Good feedback should sound like this: "You are so important to this office that I thought you should know the effects of your behavior." Put in slightly different words, "I like you, and I'm happy about what you're doing" or "I like you, but I'm unhappy with what you're doing right now." In practice, the clause reflecting the co-worker's value ("I like you") is usually not spoken, but the feeling should be clearly implied. Correcting a problem while hurting a colleague is destructive criticism. In dentistry, where therapy is designed to preserve the integrity of supporting structures, feedback should be as specific and limited as possible.

The art of giving feedback is discussed by answering four questions: (1) Which circumstances require that feedback be given? (2) When and where should feedback be given? (3) How should feedback be expressed, and (4) What should be done after feedback is offered? An additional section is devoted to feedback at chairside, where the presence of a patient requires some adjustment in what professionals say to each other. Finally, ways of responding to feedback are considered.

TO FEEDBACK OR NOT TO FEEDBACK?

Knowing which situations call for feedback and which should be ignored is the first step in giving feedback. Even a well-meaning and tactfully phrased suggestion may produce friction if it is inappropriate. King Leopold I of Belgium is supposed to have written to his niece, "I have not been able to ascertain that you have really grown taller lately, but I must recommend it strongly." As valuable as it might be to be taller and as carefully expressed as this message is, it is still unwise and poor feedback. The niece obviously had little control over changing her growth and may have been "hurt" by the implication that she is short.

Praise All Worthy Behavior

The first rule of feedback is never to miss an opportunity to recognize meritorious acts. Feeding back success builds positive self-images, improves rapport, and, more than anything else, increases chances of similar positive behaviors occurring in the future.[3] Behavior that is ignored soon disappears unless it is intrinsically maintained by pride or other values. A smile or "thank you" can often obtain results that money and coercion cannot. But care must be taken to make praise credible or both the positive feedback and the speaker may be disregarded.[4]

Negative Feedback May Be Needed

Negative feedback is appropriate to protect patients and the staff, to provide better care, and when one's integrity is being attacked. If the chairside assistant notices problems with intravenous or nitrous oxide sedation analgesia, to cite an obvious example, this should be brought to the dentist's attention. If any staff member learns of a patient who feels mistreated, they should speak up. When co-workers make unreasonable requests, feedback is needed to prevent further deterioration of communication.

Avoid Useless Feedback

Many comments are useless, unnecessary, or damaging. Accidents or apparently uncharacteristic behavior are better not commented on. Past events are also out of a person's power to control. Problems occurring because of lack of training or ability should be resolved through education or termination.[5] Finally, the person offering feedback must be recognized as having the authority to make such comments.

- *(Assistant to receptionist)* "I know you're busy now but let me just show you how to fix the problem in the day sheet." (The assistant may be right but this is not part of the assistant's job.)
- *(Dentist to hygienist)* "Why don't you use the universal scaler there?" (The dentist should be concerned about removal of calculus and freedom from trauma, not technique.)

WHEN AND WHERE SHOULD FEEDBACK BE GIVEN?

Timing and location are critical to the success of feedback. As the hangman placed the noose around the neck of the convicted killer he sternly moralized, "I hope this teaches you a lesson." The decision to respond ultimately depends on its effects on patient care.

Patient Care Is Paramount

If a dentist tells the assistant in the presence of the patient that the amalgam is not being mixed correctly, the assistant is embarrassed and the patient questions both quality of care and the judgment of a dentist who would hire an inept employee. The patient need not be present for mistimed feedback to be damaging. Patients grow irritable when waiting for staff to work out their problems. An employee who has been severely criticized immediately before seeing a patient is apt to be accident prone, inattentive, or even rude.

Timing and corrective feedback are always a trade-off. The damage to patient care caused by not making a necessary adjustment immediately must be weighed against the disruption that the feedback might cause. Many modifications can be made in the patient's presence without raising suspicions. Nonverbal cues or positive, nonjudgmental remarks ("I think we need a longer mixing time for Mrs. Boulder's amalgam.") can be used.

Nonthreatening Locations Amplify Feedback

Environments that make others defensive or embarrassed should be avoided because feelings will be a barrier to the information given. The front desk, an operatory, or the hallway is a poor location for feedback because conversations can be overheard. The dentist's personal office affords privacy but reduces other employees' status and makes them defensive. The lab or employee lounge is good neutral territory for feedback of an extensive or sensitive nature.

A Word in Time Saves Nerves

Both positive and negative comments should be made as soon as practically possible to improve accuracy and reduce chances of the mistake being repeated. Delayed criticism can become distorted by rehearsing it and bottled-up emotions are an obstacle to later communication.

When it is impossible to give immediate feedback because the location or the timing is inappropriate, an agreement can be made to talk later.

- *(Dentist to receptionist)* "Remind me that we should discuss scheduling before I leave this evening."
- *(Dentist to assistant in presence of patient)* "I've just thought of something. Let's talk about tray set-ups after lunch, okay?"

HOW SHOULD FEEDBACK BE EXPRESSED?

There are three principles of giving feedback: be concrete, be solution-oriented, and be careful of others' feelings. In the words of an anonymous wag, "Try to make your words tender; you may have to eat them."

Feedback Should Be Concrete

Consider two ways a dentist might criticize the receptionist's handling of a telephone call:

- *(Dentist to receptionist)* "You didn't ask the patient if you could help him or thank him for calling."
- *(Dentist to receptionist)* "You have a lousy telephone personality."

Only the first example contains information the receptionist can use to do a better job. The second alternative stimulates defensiveness, lowers morale, and leaves the receptionist wondering what could be done better.

Focus on Solutions

For small problems, the best feedback may mention only the desired response and omit the problem entirely. When dentists see calculus remaining on a patient's teeth they may say,

- "Mrs. Brown has those new restorations on the lower molars. Let's give her a specially thorough cleaning there."
- "There's calculus remaining on the mandibular molars and that could create a problem."

The first response suggests appropriate corrective action without fixing blame. It creates little defensiveness and is subtle enough to use in a patient's presence. The second alternative raises concerns without necessarily moving toward correcting the problem.

Defensiveness Destroys Cooperation and Rapport

The manner in which feedback is expressed is as important as what is actually said. When the words or nonverbal communication convey a feeling of judgment, control, hidden motives, lack of caring, superiority, or dogmatism, listeners typically respond by erecting defensive barriers.[6] Confusion results when the verbal and the nonverbal messages are not consistent.[7] An unexpected frown with no explanation or a suggestion followed by a shrug and "Oh, never mind" leaves the listener groping.

A general strategy that avoids defensiveness is called the "feedback sandwich." Its three parts include: (1) praise, (2) negative feedback, and (3) praise. There is no better hearing aid than a compliment. It is also wise to reaffirm the trust in a relationship after criticism has been given.

- *(Assistant to co-worker)* "Thank you for straightening up the lab last night. I was really behind. The only problem is that Dr. Forbes couldn't find the mixing bowls. Why don't we do it together and I can learn some things from you, too."
- *(Dentist to new chairside assistant)* "You're so fast and you have the ideal treatment sequence down so well. But sometimes I don't go exactly by the book, so if you'll watch me too I'm sure we'll be very efficient in no time."

WHAT SHOULD BE DONE AFTER FEEDBACK IS GIVEN?

Find Out How Feedback Is Received

If feedback is important enough to give, it is also important to make certain that it is understood and that there are no strong negative feelings preventing its implementation. Sometimes an unnatural hesitation or facial expression may signal trouble. When nonverbal reactions leave significant doubt, it is appropriate to ask, "How do you feel about this suggestion?" or "You seem uncertain about this idea."

Praise Any Approximation of Desired Behavior

After criticism has been given, it is mandatory to watch for and reward improvements. This shows that the person who offered the criticism really cares about having things done the right way. More importantly, it increases the likelihood of appropriate behavior in the future.[3] It is imprudent to withhold praise until a corrected behavior is performed perfectly. Every improvement should be commented upon because this is the fastest way to improve a skill.

Do Not Repeat Unheeded Criticism

When learning a skill, students may need a few subtle reminders. But persistent problems do not respond well to repeated criticism. Typically this signals some serious underlying problem and no progress can be made until the obstruction is discovered and removed. The situation calls for a private discussion in which assertive messages are used.

- "I am frustrated because you have not responded to my suggestions."
- "The problem I mentioned last week is persisting. This is hurting our effectiveness and I would like to talk about it."

COMMUNICATION AT CHAIRSIDE

An uninitiated observer at chairside might mistakenly conclude that little communication is taking place between dentist and assistant. Certainly very little is being said. The nonverbal communication is actually a constant, rich, varied, and specialized exchange. The predominance of nonverbals in this situation is due to the patient's presence and the need for speed, and it is made possible by the routine nature of most dental treatments.

Patients do not want to hear a constant stream of technical chatter—directives from the dentist, questions from the assistant. It is also prudent to minimize discussion of techniques (extractions and injections), instruments (clamps and drills), and conditions (exposures and bleeding) that make patients anxious. Moreover, all of this talking would take too long.

The answer is found in nonverbal communication. The basic patterns of treatment are guided and adjusted by pace, hesitation, variation in hand pressure, facial expression, gestures, and even comments to the patient to which the assistant is expected to respond ("Alright, Mrs. Palmer, we are placing the rubber dam now for this restoration").

A primary concern is patient and staff health and safety. The assistant should monitor the patient's reaction to treatment while the dentist is busy in the mouth. A gesture can draw the dentist's attention to white knuckles gripping the arms of the chair or to shallow breathing, pallor, and perspiration without alarming the patient. Occasionally, because of a difference in vantage point, the assistant may notice something of importance in the patient's mouth, unremoved caries, for example. This must be brought to the dentist's attention and can be done without worrying the patient.

- *(Chairside assistant to dentist)* "Doctor, hold your mirror so you can see the buccal cusp."

Reliance on nonverbal cues promotes essential efficiency and speed at chairside. Knowing what to expect next in the sequence of treatment reduces reaction time. But when the normal situation is altered, overanticipation causes errors and delays. For this reason, the dentist should verbally signal any change as soon as its need is recognized.

- *(Dentist to assistant)* "We definitely have pulpal involvement on the second molar."
- *(Dentist, picking up the handpiece)* "Just one more time and the preparation will be complete."

RECEIVING FEEDBACK

Ideally, all feedback would be given according to the suggestions in this chapter. Realistically, a lot of crude and ineffective criticism is encountered. Even under less than optimal circumstances, there is much that a skilled feedback "receiver" can do.[8]

Let us use the example of a dentist who complains to the receptionist, "Why are you always interrupting me with telephone calls from people I don't want to talk to? Use your judgment." This is poor feedback because it is fault-finding and too general. Nothing is said that helps the receptionist avoid the problem in the future. A skilled feedback receiver would not leave this situation without a clearer understanding of the kind of behavior needed to correct the problem. If specific solutions are not offered in the feedback, they can be suggested by the person receiving the criticism.

- *(Receptionist to dentist)* "Well, I'm confused. I don't really think I can decide for you. But I can ask the callers for the nature of their business and how urgent it is."

A type of feedback to which it is more difficult to respond involves generalized attacks on character rather than the behavior that needs correcting.[9] The natural tendency toward defensiveness can be handled by separating the behavior from the personal comment. The behavior should be dealt with first and factually. In the two examples that follow, identify the mature, constructive response. A hygienist says in disgust to the only assistant in the office, "Who's the lazy-bones who forgot to clean off the lab counters last night?"

- "I didn't forget. I was helping Dr. Quincy until after 5:30."

- "Yes, I know that's my responsibility, but I was helping Dr. Quincy until 5:30 last night."

Both responses explain the facts of the situation, but the first is combative. By acknowledging responsibility in the second example, a more constructive dialogue is invited. It may be necessary, if personal, global attacks disguised as feedback persist, to respond separately to this issue with an assertive message.

- *(Assistant to hygienist)* "It bothers me when my work is criticized without knowing all the facts. I would prefer to talk things out without blaming anyone."

Others should be rewarded when they give reasonable feedback. A prompt response, a "thank you," or a clarification of what is expected increases the likelihood of more appropriate feedback to come. Feedback need not be perfect to merit commendation.

- *(Dentist to chairside assistant)* "Thanks for letting me know the patient dislikes nitrous. Next time point to it in the chart before I start talking about it."

CASE: BEING RIGHT AND BEING HELPFUL

Polly Sharp, the new receptionist, stuck her head in the operatory where Dr. Kind was performing an endodontic procedure on Mrs. Panagotacas. "Excuse me just a minute. I need to know if Mrs. Panagotacas' work was preauthorized for insurance."

The dentist stopped and turned part way to face the receptionist. "I believe Sue did that before she left. If the work is not in the chart, you might check the 'pending file'."

"Oh, I looked everywhere. This thing's a mess and we need some sort of organization so we don't have these problems," continued the receptionist.

Now the dentist turned around completely to face the staff member and said, "Mrs. Panagotacas' work is completely covered by insurance. I'm glad you're working on the insurance processing and I'd like to talk with you specifically about this at 4:30 this afternoon." His voice was pleasant but slow and firm. As soon as he finished speaking, he smiled then quickly turned to resume treatment of the patient.

At four-thirty, when no one was at the front desk except for Polly, Dr. Kind came out and sat down. "I appreciate your concern about the insurance system. You're very perceptive to recognize that it needs a lot of work.

"But I also have to give you some feedback about patient care here. When with a patient, I want to devote my full attention to them, so I should only be interrupted for serious problems that can't wait. It is also a good practice to keep financial matters out of the operatory.

"I know you're eager to get started organizing this front desk. That's one of the reasons I hired you. Now let's see what you have come up with. . . ."

ANALYSIS

In this example, the receptionist was right in what she had to say, but she created obstacles for herself by the way she proceeded. The dentist did not need to be told that problems exist; he already knows. The greatest miscalculation was in timing and location. Dr. Kind had to remind Polly that patient care comes first. The comment that "things are a mess and need some sort of organization" is too general to be of help and is fault-finding rather than pointing to a solution.

The contrast in this example is the dentist's use of a "feedback sandwich." He dissipates defensiveness by praising what was appropriate in the employee's behavior. His suggested behavior is solution-oriented and concrete, and he reaffirms the receptionist's worth after offering a criticism. A timely response was prevented by his first responsibility to the patient, but he handled this by naming a definite time to attend to the issue. The receptionist was put at ease by meeting on her own "turf" with no audience.

Dr. Kind also reacted appropriately to the receptionist's ill-considered feedback. He acknowledged what was true in her remarks and set a later time to address in specific detail all of her concerns.

REFERENCES

1. Maltz, M. *Psycho-cybernetics.* New York: Pocket Books, 1970.
2. Wiener, N. *The human use of human beings: Cybernetics and society.* New York: Avon, 1954.
3. Skinner, B.F. *Science and human behavior.* New York: Macmillan, 1953.
4. Bergin, A.E. The effects of dissonant persuasive communications upon changes in self-referring attitude. *Journal of Personality,* 1962, 30, 423.
5. Mager, R.F., & Pipe, P. *Analyzing performance problems, or "you really oughta wana."* Belmont, Calif.: Fearon, 1970.

6. Gibb, J.R. Defensive communication. *Journal of Communication*, 1964, 11, 141.
7. Satir, V. *Peoplemaking*. Palo Alto, Calif.: Science and Behavior, 1972.
8. Simon, S.B. *Negative criticism: Its swath of destruction and what to do about it*. Niles, Ill.: Argus Communications, 1978.
9. Smith, M.J. *When I say no, I feel guilty*. New York: Dial Books, 1975.

EXERCISES

15–1. In the following case, identify the guidelines for good feedback that have been ignored. There are at least six.

> It is quarter to six. The receptionist, chairside assistant, and dentist are putting on their coats at the front desk. The receptionist says to the assistant, "Gail, you still haven't told me whether you can drive Pam and me to Cleveland on Saturday." Gail answers, somewhat in a huff, "Oh, gee. I'm not sure. I just haven't had time to think about it. I've got to go. I'll let you know," and she starts toward the door. Dr. Pratt interrupts, "Hey, wait a minute, Gail. You've been awfully wound up this week. You'd better settle down and not be so huffy with Ann. And while I'm thinking about it, you were pretty short with Mrs. Pollick the day before yesterday, too. I don't like that and I expect you to do something about it. Do you understand?" There was a long silence. Dr. Pratt said, "Okay, good," and left.

15–2. Prepare a feedback script. Identify three specific situations that have been annoying you. Make certain that each is a case involving the care of patients or harmony in the office and that the person causing the problem can change his or her behavior. Write the problem behavior at the top of a page. Place the following headings along the left margin: Preserve patient care, nonthreatening location, timing, concrete description, solution, reduce defensiveness, check understanding, praise positive behavior. Write notes to yourself beside each heading. Rehearse your script alone or with a friend. Deliver the feedback as you have rehearsed it and watch what happens to your own self-esteem and to office efficiency.

15–3. Make a list of the differences between the communication during dental treatment and the communication around an operating table in a hospital. Next list the similarities. What is the reason for the differences?

15–4. Comment on the three responses offered in the situation below. A dentist watches as a difficult patient is rude to the receptionist and leaves abruptly. The dentist says, "You've got a lot to learn about human nature. Can't you tell when a patient is trying to get out of paying a bill?"

The receptionist responds:

a. "How can you tell how bright I am?"

b. "I guess it might have looked like that, but Mrs. Bently did pay."

c. "When you question my judgment, particularly in front of other patients, I get upset and worried about what patients might think. It would be easier for me if you just asked specific questions, like 'Has Mrs. Bently paid?' and that will help me do my job better."

DISCUSSION OF EXERCISES

15–1. This example shows how to break almost every rule in the book simultaneously. The dentist should have stayed out of the personal situation between Gail and Ann. But he should have spoken up as soon as the patient left. Criticizing the assistant in the presence of the receptionist is tactless. The feedback is ineffective because it is negative and too general. No follow-up is planned. Different readings of this case can probably uncover further problems.

15–2. Sample feedback script for situation where dentist runs fingers through hair before examining a patient: (1) preserve patient care—no direct reference in front of patient, (2) nonthreatening location—in dentist's office, (3) timing—at end of day, (4) concrete description—"Mr. Dickter looked at you sorta funny today when you examined him after running your fingers through your hair. I have noticed that a couple of times." (5) concrete solution—"As a signal, why don't I just hold the mirror and explorer until you wash. That won't even be noticed by the patient." (6) reduce defensiveness—comment on value of rapport, (7) check understanding—get dentist to paraphrase solution agreed upon, (8) praise positive behavior—big smile when hands are washed.

15–3. *Differences:* The hospital setting involves more gross body movement such as coming and going with more verbal communication; more informal, personal, and emotional discussion; and repetition of critical requests to ensure accuracy of understanding. *Similarities:* Less work-related directions given to better trained and more experienced workers and freedom to correct the doctor regarding problems that affect patient health. The major difference is presence of a conscious patient in dentistry. This is a source of stress that can be reduced by effective communication skills.

15–4. **a.** Defensive reaction focusing on one's own personality not the problem that needs mending.

b. A proper response which states the facts and acknowledges some value in what the critical dentist said.

c. An appropriate assertive response of the DESC script type. Describe problem behavior ("When you question"), express feelings ("I get upset"), specify desired behavior ("It would be easier for me . . ."), and consequences ("that would help").

16

Intraoffice Communication

Office policy and a hardworking staff do not eliminate the need for communication among co-workers. Constant adjustments are required to keep an office running effectively because of changes in procedures, patients, turnover, and growth and education of the staff and the dentist.

In this chapter we focus on staff meetings. The typical image of a meeting includes a group sitting around a table discussing topics. This chapter is also about "informal meetings," such as the dentist telling the staff one by one about a new policy or several staff members casually discussing a problem and agreeing on a plan. Timing, attendance, participation, and location are structural characteristics of meetings that are less important than the functional aspects of (1) sharing information and (2) reaching group decisions. Some of the major ways good meetings promote practice efficiency and effectiveness include creating common expectations, reducing the need for individual feedback, permitting negative feedback without embarrassing individuals, and enhancing quality decision making and morale though participation.[1–3]

Both formal and informal meetings combine information dissemination and problem solving.[4] They frequently include "hidden agenda" items involving social and status needs of participants, as well. The discussion in this chapter is simplified by describing the features of information meetings and problem solving meetings separately.

INFORMATION MEETINGS

The most common functions of staff meetings are to present information and elicit feedback. In this format, the dentist generally makes announcements or presents new policy and invites reaction. This structure appears suited to dentists' needs for efficiency, solution orientation, and control. Three suggestions are offered that can improve such meetings.

First, when new policies are announced, it is prudent to begin with a history of the problem and to mention alternatives that have been considered.[5] If these steps are omitted, the new policy may appear arbitrary, no matter how brilliant the solution. For example, the dentist might review the problems the office has had with collections. Alternatives such as collection agencies, cash discounts, and "aggressive front office tactics" would be discussed. When the "cash basis" system is announced as the new policy, it will be both meaningful and plausible.

Second, the dentist should avoid open-ended discussion of new policy. Instead, each staff member in turn should be asked to explain the impact of the policy on his or her job. This gives a reading on potential implementation problems and is a means of verifying that the policy is clear. Staff who do not understand how a "cash basis" system functions are unlikely to respond to the vague invitation, "Well, what do you think?" If each must describe the impact of the new system, both understanding and real obstacles will be revealed.

A third practice that can strengthen information meetings is to invite each staff member to share individual accomplishments and concerns by calling on each in succession. These will come out selectively and informally in office "gossip." Having a common forum is more productive.

- *(Dentist to staff)* "I've been talking about what is important to me for a while now. I'd like to hear some of what is on each of your minds. Everybody will get a chance. So tell me what do you think has been going really well for you since the last time and what are the problems? Let's start with Jan."

The same three suggestions mentioned for improving an information meeting apply to a weekly staff meeting attended by all employees or a "rolling" meeting where the dentist contacts individual staff members in sequence. When a formal meeting is used, it is helpful to hold it regularly, to make it short (perhaps 15 minutes), to end *exactly* on time, avoid staff time such as lunch hours, and to postpone any unfinished business until the next regularly scheduled meeting or obtain consensus that a special meeting is necessary.

PROBLEM SOLVING MEETINGS

Meetings to solve common problems are difficult to manage but they can be very rewarding. Vacation schedules, dress standards, work assignments, policy for handling emergencies or problem patients, recall systems, records, and care of equipment are all examples of issues that might be considered by the entire office staff. The general rule is that anyone affected by a problem or its solution should have input in solving it.

Anyone involved with such meetings must have been frustrated at times when "no one sticks to the topic." If permitted, personal digressions and petty concerns tend to occupy much of a meeting's time. This is a natural phenomenon that must be understood before suggesting management tactics (Table 16–1).[6]

Need for Acceptance

Individuals use groups for four purposes: personal acceptance, exchange of information, resolution of group problems, and attempted control over others.[7] Of these, the primary motive is personal acceptance. Those who do not feel valued withdraw from exchanging information and do not contribute to problem solving. This can be a source of frustration for goal-oriented high achievers, and a balance must be struck between the task and

TABLE 16–1. OBSTACLES TO GROUP DECISION MAKING

Obstacle	Effective Management
Staff needs for personal acceptance	Acknowledge feelings Balance social and task orientation
Hidden agendas	State common agenda in concrete terms Allow some expression of hidden agendas at beginning Focus on issues, not personalities Draw out reluctant individuals
Excessive manager (dentist) control	Clearly articulate criteria for successful problem solution Delegate meeting chair to another (optional)

social functions in meetings or ultimately the solutions will be of poor quality.

Hidden Agendas

Unannounced personal expectations for the outcome of the meeting are called "hidden agendas."[8] Everyone present at a meeting may have different hidden agendas. These may include "having my solution accepted," "showing the hygienist up as being domineering," "proving to the dentist how loyal I am," or "convincing the staff that the dentist really understands what is going on at the front desk." Such hidden agendas tend to conflict with each other and are often at odds with the stated purpose of the meeting.

A skillful leader can do four things to minimize the damage caused by hidden agendas. First, the central problem should be stated in concrete terms, with public agreement obtained that this is to be the common agenda item for the meeting. "We have a very important problem that must be resolved today." A second helpful tactic is to let group members air their hidden agendas in the preliminary stages of the meeting. Sometimes the leader can recognize staff concerns without changing the common agenda. "Right, Ethel, we do need to talk about the problem with the old instruments, but right now our concern is to decide who will sterilize the instruments." The third strategy for neutralizing hidden agendas in group problem solving is to insist that discussion remain on the problem and not on the personality or relative status of staff. "Let's leave personalities out of this and try to concentrate on finding a solution we can all live with." Finally, it is helpful to ask staff members who appear reticent to explain the reasons for their hesitation. "Jay, you seem uncertain; why is that?"

Excessive Manager Control

A dentist's desire to retain control over meetings can also be an obstacle to effective problem solving. Wanting to be in charge is understandable in view of the fact that dentists are ethically, legally, and financially responsible for the acts of the entire staff insofar as they relate to dentistry. But some dentists think control means making all the decisions and doing all the work. This tends to be a burden for dentists at the same time it limits group creativity and leaves the dentist with the double task of first finding the solution then having to "sell" it. Chapter 13 may be reviewed for reasons why participation in problem solving leads to commitment and follow-through.

An alternative strategy places the leader in a position of outlining the problem and characteristics of the desired solution, then turning the talents of the staff loose to solve the problem.[5]

- *(Dentist to staff)* "I'm not particular about how the recall system operates as long as it takes no more time or paperwork than what we now have, that anybody can tell the status of a patient at a glance, and that one person is in charge. Oh, and I would like to see the patient flow up, too. The results are what I am interested in and since you people have been dealing with this on a daily basis, I'm turning to you for ideas."

In this example, the dentist has established the parameters of a successful solution and, of course, has veto power over any suggested solution that does not meet these standards. This frees the creative and participatory energies of the staff to work on the problem without having to second guess the boss. It also sets the example for the staff of exposing hidden agendas and defining acceptable solutions as distinct from individual personal preferences. More than one solution that meets all standards may be found. Staff are more willing to compromise in attacking difficult problems because all cards are already on the table and because it is understood that the dentist can impose a solution if the staff fails to agree.

CASE: GETTING EVERYONE TO COME TO THE SAME MEETING

Dr. Tagnotti, Pam (chairside), Paul (reception), and Alice (general assistant) were sitting in the lounge waiting to start a staff meeting. Paul leaned forward, impatient, "Let's get started. Pauline (the part-time hygienist) is always late anyway, and she can catch up."

Dr. Tagnotti answered, "No, I would prefer to wait because this involves everybody equally."

Pam sighed heavily and the dentist made small talk with the reluctant staff until Pauline arrived. She apologized and sat down.

The dentist began: "I am disturbed by some problems I see in office communication. What is natural and easy for you, Paul and Pam, because you have been here for several years, is still confusing for Alice and Pauline. All of us need your help because we are judged by the patients as a total practice and any inconsistency, discourtesy, or problem reflects on all of us. Personnel policies are not my long suit and I don't enjoy patching up little squabbles. I certainly won't be put in a position of having to choose favorites.

"What I want is a smooth-running office; one that is efficient and where patients and all of us enjoy being here. If that isn't everybody's primary objective, we may have to make personnel adjustments. If it is what we all want, then we should be able to work out whatever is necessary to achieve that kind of teamwork.

"I'm willing to work on this problem as long as it appears productive and as long as we can avoid personal attacks on each other. I have expressed my views about what I think we need to do. I'd like to hear from each of you in turn whether you think there is a problem and, if so, what kind of resolution you're looking for. Pam?"

Pam hesitated and looked at Paul. He was ready with an answer. "Well, naturally, we all want things to go better. But I think we can save a lot of time if we just make sure everybody knows their job and then does it. Like, look at Pauline, she can't even keep track of charts."

Pauline answered calmly, "Yes, I did have to apologize to Alice for not giving her that Palmer kid's records. But I would like to give Dr. Tagnotti's idea a try. I think there's a lot more to dentistry than can ever be put in an office manual. Like how can you anticipate how to get that 400-pound Mr. Oscar in and out of the chair?"

General laughter; then Pam volunteered, "See, we're already off the topic, aren't we?"

ANALYSIS

This dentist is handling a difficult problem very well. He has identified lack of communication as a problem that belongs to and affects the entire office and has invited all to share in its solution. An attempt to impose a solution in a situation such as this would likely fail. He has set sound ground rules for the problem's solution.

Paul has not accepted the problem yet and no progress will be possible until he does. He offers criticism of the hygienist but Pauline correctly acknowledges her behavior while turning away the personal attack with good humor.

We would respond to Pam's question ("Aren't we off the topic?") by saying "no." At least the staff is now talking with each other about things that they believe are important and have probably wanted to talk about for some time.

REFERENCES

1. Morton, J.C., Clark, J., Adelson, R., & Hornsby, J.L. *Dental teamwork strategies: Interpersonal and organizational approaches*. St. Louis: C.V. Mosby, 1980.

2. Patton, B.R., & Giffin, K. *Decision-making group interaction* (2nd ed.). New York: Harper & Row, 1978.
3. Schein, E.H. *Process consultation: Its role in organizational development.* Reading, Mass.: Addison-Wesley, 1969.
4. Townsend, R. *Up the organization: How to stop the corporation from stifling people and strangling profits.* Greenwich, Conn.: Fawcett, 1970.
5. Doyle, M., & Straus, D. *The new interaction method: How to make meetings work.* Chicago: Playboy Press, 1976.
6. Finkel, C. *Professional guide to successful meetings.* Boston: Herman Publication, 1976.
7. Gibb, J.R. Defensive communication. *Journal of Communication*, 1964, 11, 141.
8. Verderber, R.F. *Communicate* (2nd ed.). Belmont, Calif.: Wadsworth, 1978.

EXERCISES

16–1. Assume you are the dentist trying to solve a problem with the recall system. You see the hygienist alone for a minute, briefly explain what you think the problem is (the current tracking system is too cumbersome and therefore not used systematically), and outline what you would like to see in an acceptable solution. The hygienist listens and nods in apparent understanding, then jumps in with the following comment: "Right, I agree with you that Sharon (the front desk person assigned to this job) is really irresponsible. I don't think we'll get anywhere until we can get someone else in there who knows what's going on." What should you respond?

After you have made your answer above, assume that the hygienist continues, "Well, it looks like you're going to take her side no matter what. I don't know why you ask for my advice if you're not going to follow it." What should you respond now?

16–2. In your office there is a senior dentist and an associate, two part-time hygienists, a chairside assistant, a part-time floating assistant, a receptionist, and a part-time person responsible for insurance. The senior dentist decides to change all insurance claims to a universal claim form, announces this change by explaining the benefits to the associate and the two front desk staff members, and briefly notes the differences between the old and the new forms. He then asks what each person thinks of the new idea. Everyone shrugs and mumbles, "Okay, we'll try," so the dentist says "good" and walks away. How could this change be better communicated?

16–3. Think of meetings you have had at work, school, or in some other setting. Identify one group with whom you meet and list the group's name at the top of the page. In one column list the things you like best about these meetings. In another column list what you like least. Positive feedback will help insure the continuance of the things you like. Can you explain what reward people are getting for doing the things you dislike?

DISCUSSION OF EXERCISES

16–1. Two people exchanging information or trying to reach a decision constitute a meeting. It might be wise to hold a "serial" meeting with one staff member at a time if there is fear that some people will be inhibited in a larger context. But the same rules apply whether the meeting takes place once for all or is spread across several occasions. In this example, the dentist is clear about the agenda and the criteria for a solution. The hygienist seems to have a hidden agenda—to attack the receptionist. The dentist may insist that the hygienist stay on the topic, "I see you are upset about Sharon, but the problem is really to figure out how to handle recalls." Alternatively, the dentist might choose to bring out the hygienist's hidden agenda since it appears in this staff member's mind to be part of the problem. In doing this, the dentist would want to repeat the importance of the original agenda, "I want to hear your feelings about Sharon. But let's keep this in the context of the original issue of the recall system."

The hygienist's second statement can be interpreted as asking to be excused from the meeting because the hygienist does not feel accepted. This calls for restating the agenda and the dentist's role prior to exploring why the hygienist feels unaccepted. "No, wait! I'm just trying to gather information so I can make a good decision here. I'm not trying to take sides. It is obvious that you have some pretty strong feelings in general about Sharon, so let's talk about that as a separate issue either now or later this afternoon."

16–2. There are three problems here and two missed opportunities. There is no history or rationale for the change, so it appears arbitrary. Because it is presented as an accomplished fact, those present are unlikely to respond seriously to the invitation, "What do you think?" The third problem is failure to include the hygienist and perhaps the assistants, who should probably know something about the change. The opportunity is missed to find out how well each person understands the change or what obstacles exist to its implementation. This can be learned by asking for a run-through of the changes the employees see. It would also have helped to learn how the staff was doing in general at that time.

Being open to their concerns makes them open to the dentist's.

16–3. Meetings, for information or for decisions, of the whole or individual, follow all the dynamics of interpersonal relations in general. One of the most effective means of bringing meetings in line with the ideals stated in this chapter is to reward desirable behavior and withhold reward for inappropriate actions. The feedback techniques in Chapter 15 are valuable in this regard and may be used by all staff members whether or not they are "responsible" for organizing the meeting.

17

Using the Telephone Effectively

The way the telephone is used can make or break a practice. The first contact between new patients and the dental office is almost always by telephone. Many patients choose dentists based on location by looking in the telephone book. The telephone provides continuity of care by permitting a dentist to check on postoperative patients and facilitating patients' emergency care. It allows for consultation with other dentists and physicians and for credit and insurance status checks. Supplies can be ordered and all manner of professional business transacted by telephone.

The telephone is also a major source of stress. Interruptions, calls making demands, those bringing disagreeable news and solicitations are examples of uninvited intrusions into our professional lives. It is universal practice, for example, to interrupt a personal conversation to answer the ringing phone, without even knowing who is calling. Most of our lives, we are within telephone range of everyone we know and everyone who wants something of us.

INCOMING CALLS

Seven Hints on Technique for Answering the Phone

ANSWER PROMPTLY. Prevent callers from wondering about the efficiency of the office. Answer promptly: waiting increases anxiety and anger.

BE PREPARED. It is essential to have paper and pencil near the telephone in order to record information accurately. When talking to a patient-of-record, the chart should always be pulled. It may be necessary to answer specific questions or to note details of the conversation. Having the chart available, particularly if it contains a photograph or other descriptive data, will make the telephone conversation more personal.

USE NAMES. Names are wonderful for building rapport because they show a willingness to relate on an individual basis. When persons answering the telephone mention the dentist's name and their own, they signal that the office treats people as individuals and they invite the caller to do likewise.

- *(Receptionist answering the telephone)* "Hello. Drs. Armitage and Preston. This is Ann Childs."
- *(Receptionist answering the telephone)* "Good afternoon. This is Gail Lu at Dr. O'Hara's office. May I help you?"

"Doctors office" is quick and impersonal, and that is the impression callers are apt to form of offices where the telephone is answered in this fashion. Time must be taken to pronounce clearly the names of the dentists. Most first-time callers are expecting to hear only the name of the dentist they have been referred to. Group practice arrangements might be listed in the phone book to minimize this surprise.

OFFER TO HELP. The individual about to answer a ringing telephone knows something about the person on the other end even before touching the receiver. People make phone calls because they need something. Sometimes it is the need to make, change, or cancel an appointment. Perhaps it is a problem with medications or questions about payment for services. Maybe it is an invitiation to speak at Rotary or a request to buy an extra quart of milk on the way home. Regardless of what is actually said when answering the phone, the feeling conveyed must always be "how can I help you."[1] The most common blend of emotions in patients calling the dental office is uncertainty and hopefulness, usually tinged with traces of defensiveness.[2] Everything that can be done to dissipate these unpleasant emotions aids communication and creates a positive impression of the practice. A pleasant telephone manner and a warm and supporting response to requests are powerful practice builders.

KNOW OFFICE POLICY. It is imperative that any person answering the telephone know the office policies. Examples of cases where the office help must be consistent with office practices include information about first appointments, fees, responding to emergencies and patients who are "shopping around," and knowing when the dentist or hygienist should be called to the telephone. Credibility in the practice suffers when patients are told "I'm new; I don't know about that yet," or when they are given misinformation.

HELP CALLERS WHO HAVE PROBLEMATIC REQUESTS. It is usually possible to offer help and show concern for callers even when it is impossible to comply literally with their requests. Table 17–1 shows several questions and situations where it is hard or unwise to respond literally or immediately. Examples of both inappropriate and helpful remarks are listed. The helpful response always begins by giving a reason or by stating what *can* be done prior to rejecting the request.

INFORM CALLERS WHEN THEY ARE INTERRUPTING. Answering two calls at the same time or coordinating calls and patients in the office requires a good memory, judgment, and tact. Table 17–2 shows the typical pattern of dealing with multiple calls.

There are a few exceptions to this basic pattern when judgment and clear office policy are helpful. Emergencies should not be put "on hold." This is why it is important to ask and wait for a reply before putting a caller on hold. Some individuals prefer to ask the second caller the nature of their business before deciding how to proceed. No caller should ever be put off for the personal convenience of the person answering the telephone.

Answering Services versus Answering Machines

Offices are closed during lunch hour, on certain days of the week, and for vacations. Practices must deal with calls during this time and with emergency care for patients-of-record at any time it is required.[3] Professional answering services are the preferred means of dealing with these situations. Individuals who work for such firms are experienced in proper telephone techniques and can convey an impression of caring even when the dentist is not immediately available. They can also exercise some discretion in the case of emergencies.

Answering machines are more impersonal than an answering

TABLE 17–1. INAPPROPRIATE AND HELPFUL RESPONSES TO PROBLEMATIC QUESTIONS

Request	Inappropriate Response	Helpful Response
"What would it cost to have a small filling?" (Inappropriate question)	"I cannot answer that."	"Dr. Doyle always discusses fees and treatment options prior to beginning work. But it might be misleading to quote prices over the telephone without knowing your individual needs. Can we schedule . . .?
(Patient at desk or on other line)	"Doctor's office. Will you hold?" (click without waiting for an answer)	"This is Alice Gervosky in Dr. Thompson's office. I am with a patient. Do you mind if I put you on hold for just a minute?" (wait for answer)
"How long has it been since I had my bridge put in?" (Information not immediately available)	"I don't know. No one here can help you right now."	I'm sure that the information is in the records, but it will take a few minutes to locate it. Can I call you back?"
"I really need to see the doctor before I go on vacation." (Difficult request)	"Oh, I don't know. I'm not sure we can help you on such short notice."	"Yes, I'll get you in as soon as possible. Let me look . . ."
"My son is sick. I'll have to cancel. (Disappointing or inconvenient information)	"Well if you really can't make it . . ."	"I'm sorry to hear that Jimmy is sick and I can see why you would want to stay at home this afternoon."
(Dentist not available)	"He cannot come to the telephone right now."	"Dr. Brightner is with a patient. Perhaps I can help you."

service and are restricted in two-way communication. Thus, every effort should be made in their use to add animation and personalization of voice (without sounding unprofessional) and to anticipate callers' needs. An explanation of office hours and assurance of emergency care and a prompt response are helpful at the beginning of the taped message. It is useful to review several months' inquiries from patients to determine whether brief recorded infor-

TABLE 17–2. HANDLING MULTIPLE CALLS OR PATIENTS IN THE OFFICE

First Call or Patient	Second Call or Patient
(Excuse yourself) "I'm sorry; there is a call on the other line. I will put you on hold and then I'll be right back."	(Answer call and explain the situation) "Dr. Barlow's office. Good morning; this is Peggy. I am with a patient. Do you mind if I put you on hold for a minute?" (You must wait for an answer) "Okay."
(Transact business) "Thank you for waiting, Mr. Thompson . . ."	(Return to caller) Thank you for being so patient. How can I help you?"
Exceptions	
Reason	**Action**
When asked if you can "put him or her on hold," the second caller announces an acute emergency	Promise to handle and ask first caller or patient to wait
Second caller states desire to speak to someone else	Transfer or take message
Anticipate a lengthy or important conversation with first caller or patient	Ask if second caller can be handled first or take second caller's telephone number and call back

mation can handle some of the more common concerns. Machines that limit the length of a patient's message can be frustrating.

An example of a pleasant, concise, and helpful recorded message is as follows:

> "Hello. Dr. Gaber's office is closed until Monday. The office will be open at 8 o'clock Monday morning. If you have an emergency, you can contact Dr. Gaber at 491-9313. If you wish to leave a message, at the tone, state your name, telephone number, and message. Thank you."

Regardless of whether a service or machine is used, messages should be collected frequently and patient requests attended to promptly. It is also helpful to see periodically what impression patients receive by telephoning the service or machine yourself.

Taking Messages

Messages are second-hand communication between two people who want to talk with each other. Accuracy and completeness are the essential ingredients of a message that meets the needs of both parties, and the person taking the information must convey an impression of competence and willingness to help.

COMPLETE MESSAGES SAVE TIME. Table 17–3 illustrates the seven components of a good telephone message. The date and time, often overlooked, are important and sometimes may indicate whether the call needs to be returned at all. The caller's name is crucial, and it is a good policy to ask callers to spell their names if there is any doubt. Phone numbers, including area codes if different, should be repeated. Most callers do not mind spending a few extra seconds to ensure that their name and number are correct. They are usually impressed by the caring and attention to detail. The person taking the message should inquire about the caller's needs. For example, the receptionist might say, "Dr. Palmer is seeing patients at City General this morning and he should be back by noon. Is there anything I can help you with?" or "I will ask Dr. Palmer to return your call about noon when he comes back. What should I tell him you are calling about?"

Information about the purpose of a call can be a tremendous timesaver for the dentist and will certainly make the office look efficient. Often the caller's needs can be dealt with by the person taking the message. Patients may ask to speak with the dentist about matters such as payments, changing appointments, and emergencies, items that a qualified receptionist can handle quite effectively.

- *(Receptionist to patient)* "Yes, I can tell you about your outstanding balance, Mr. Conklin."

It would also be appropriate to make a note in the patient record. In the case of Mr. Conklin, it might say, "Pt called 4–12 at 4 asking what he still owes on bridge. Told $450, but he should have

TABLE 17–3. EXAMPLE OF A COMPLETE TELEPHONE MESSAGE

Item	Example
Date and time	Wed 11/10 9:20
Person called	Dr. Palmer
Caller (background)	Dr. Wiseman at City General
Caller's need	Wants opinion on impactions of Jerry Nelson (chart attached)
Call back number	212-7900, ext 36
Call back instructions	Can reach him between 1 and 2. Otherwise he will call again after 4:00 today
Name or initials of person taking message	DWC

paid all but $300 by now. Seems upset. His final appointment is Friday."

Messages that prepare the dentist in advance for calling back create a professional impression. If the dentist is expected to return a call, it is also helpful to arrange a convenient time. "Dr. Palmer should be free about noon. Would that be a convenient time for him to return your call?" It is less desirable to ask the caller when it would be convenient to call back, as this implies a promise the dentist may not be able to keep. If the caller prefers to call again, the person taking the message should suggest suitable times. "Dr. Palmer will be with patients until about 4:30. On Thursday he will be at the VA Hospital all day."

Putting Calls Through

Policies should be set and discussed concerning the circumstances under which the dentist may be interrupted and called to the telephone. Implementing such a policy will still require discretion and skill on the part of the receptionist. If there is doubt, the following approach can be tried.

- *(Receptionist to caller)* "Dr. Delmost will be with patients for the next hour and a half. Is this something that can wait until then?"

When interrupting the dentist, there should be no doubt in the mind of the patient being treated regarding the professional nature of the interruption. The receptionist should explain the nature of the call and ask what the dentist wishes to do.

Anticipating Incoming Calls

Some calls can be anticipated by the dentist. Warning the receptionist of these in advance can improve performance and the image of the office.

- *(Dentist to receptionist)* "Sometime today I'm expecting a call from Dr. Mussleman about Paul Dolson's daughter's impactions and a call from the University about a continuing education course. On the course, just ask them whether there is a discount because of my teaching and then make out a check for the amount they say."

This will save time for the caller, the receptionist, and the dentist. It will also create a favorable impression when the receptionist answers, "Oh yes, Dr. Mussleman. Dr. Jackson was expecting your call."

Explain When People Are Unavailable

When the caller asks for someone who is unavailable, tact must be used to avoid unflattering impressions of the office as a whole. Table 17–4 shows several examples of appropriate and inappropriate responses when the person requested by the caller is not available. It is necessary to give a reason why the requested person is unavailable, and something should be said or suggested about when they will be available and an offer of help made. For this system to work effectively, the receptionist must be familiar with the office routine and the regular personal schedules of the staff. Anything unusual or the need to leave the office should be brought to the receptionist's attention.

OUTGOING CALLS

Using the Telephone to Extend the Practice

The telephone can be used effectively to reduce the number of broken appointments by reminding patients a day or two in advance of their scheduled time. When such calls are made, it is useful to have the chart available. Patients may have questions and the chart makes the patient easier to visualize, which in turn results in a more personal call. Many offices use charts with a conspicuous place for the patient's home and work telephone num-

TABLE 17–4. INAPPROPRIATE AND APPROPRIATE WAYS OF SAYING THAT SOMEONE IS NOT AVAILABLE

Request	Inappropriate Response	Appropriate Response
"I want to talk to the dentist."	"He is busy right now."	"He's with a patient. Is there someone else who can help you?"
"Is the dentist there?"	"He's not here today."	"Dr. Margosian does not work on Thursdays. He will be in tomorrow. Can you tell me what you are calling about?"
"Can I talk to Don?"	"He went down to the store for something."	"Don is out of the office on an errand. He should be back by 3:30. Can I have him call you?"

bers. Next to these numbers should be space for adding important personal information. Phonetic spelling of difficult names, works nights, hard of hearing, parents' last name if different from child's, are examples.

The dentist can also use the telephone as a rapport and practice builder. A brief call to postsurgical patients or ones who have had extensive work done requires only a few minutes at the end of the day before the charts are filed. Calling to find out how a new denture is fitting or to reinforce instructions shows concern and may save time later correcting a problem or avoiding an interruption.

Preparing to Make Calls

When making outgoing calls, you should give all the information you would expect if you were taking a message. Your first sentence should contain three items of information: (1) name of the person making the call, (2) name of the person with whom you wish to speak, and (3) the purpose of the call. For example, in placing a call to a patient, the receptionist might say, "Hello, Mrs. Baker? This is Kathy Ching in Dr. Downy's office and I am calling about your appointment on Thursday." A dentist telephoning a colleague might say, "Hi. This is Dr. James and I'd like to talk with Dr. Pennypacker about some dental society business if he is not with a patient." When calling for the dentist, enough information should be given to determine whether an interruption is warranted. If a return call is possible, this can be mentioned. When calling about medical conditions or for other professional information, the answers should be recorded in the chart and a confirming letter requested.

Telephone companies recommend that executives place their own calls directly, not through the receptionist.[4] This is faster, avoids miscommunication, and conveys personal interest. When telephoning long distance, this should be stated in the first sentence in order to avoid being put on an expensive hold.

- *(Dentist to secretary of state society)* "Good morning, this is Dr. Farnsworth in San Diego. I am calling for Barbara Ruddy to discuss the workshop at the March meeting."

Offices require policies that cover personal calls. It is customary to have two lines for incoming calls and one for outgoing ones. Almost all offices discourage the receipt of personal calls at work. Most also do not allow personal calls to be made during working hours, or limit these to necessities, such as car repairs.

CASE: QUICK AND INEFFICIENT TELEPHONE TECHNIQUE

A patient telephones, identifying herself as Sheila Person, and asks to speak to the dentist. The receptionist explains that the dentist is with a patient and asks whether the doctor can call back. The receptionist takes the caller's number and leaves a message.

Dr. Pablos finishes her surgery an hour later and stops by the front desk. She sees the note, "Phone Sheila Person—624-3372," and asks the receptionist who this is and what was wanted. The employee does not know.

At lunch the dentist calls, but there is no answer. She tries later that afternoon and is told that the caller is the wife of a patient named Basil Morrison and that she wants an itemized list of the work performed before she will pay the bill. The dentist scowls and answers, "Yes, I remember that case, but I'll have to ask my receptionist to pull your husband's chart and let you know the exact figures." The dentist hands the telephone to the receptionist and marches back to her office.

By saving a few seconds or not wanting to appear too forward when the original call came in, the receptionist wasted the dentist's and the patient's time and caused some embarrassment for the office.

REFERENCES

1. Reynolds, H., & Tramel, M.E. *Executive time management.* Englewood Cliffs, New Jersey: Prentice-Hall, 1979.
2. Froelich, R.E., Bishop, F.M., & Dworkin, S.F. *Communication in the dental office: A programmed manual for the dental professional.* St Louis: C.V. Mosby, 1976.
3. American Dental Association. *ADA principles of ethics and code of professional conduct.* Chicago: American Dental Association, undated.
4. Engstrom, R.T., & MacKenzie, R.A. *Managing your time: Practical guidelines on the effective use of time.* Grand Rapids, Mi.: Zondervan, 1967.

EXERCISES

17–1. Reread the case above. Describe how you would handle the situation. If a message is appropriate, write one. If you would interrupt Dr. Pablos, decide what you would say.

17–2. Three awkward types of telephone calls are listed below. Construct a messsage suitable for each.

a. Patient cancels with little warning for second time.

b. Patient telephones to warn you he will not be able to pay for the crown that is to be delivered today.

c. Patient insists on an immediate appointment for a non-emergency situation.

17–3. Telephone the phone company and ask what courses or written materials are available on telephone technique.

17–4. Prepare three 3 × 5 cards that read, "You have very pleasant phone manners." Place the cards beside your telephone and when you speak with someone who has good telephone manners, tell him or her. Then turn over the card and write down the details of the conversation that were so impressive to you.

DISCUSSION OF EXERCISES

17–1. Never miss a chance to help both the caller and the dentist. Ask if you can help Sheila Person. If there is hesitancy on the part of the caller, you may wish to say, "Can I tell Dr. Pablos what this is about?" This latter question will often uncover something that can be dealt with by the receptionist. The situation in this case should never get to the message or interruption stage.

17–2. Many different messages are appropriate. These situations call for some assertiveness as well as offering to help, within reason:

a. I'm sorry to hear that your son is sick again. That must be hard on you. But it also denies another patient the dentist's time when you give us so little warning."

b. "Thank you for the advanced notice. Let's see what alternatives we can come up with."

c. "I understand your need. Let me go to the book and see what the very first opening is."

17–3. Local telephone companies often conduct training seminars or know where they can be found. There are also pamphlets available. This can be a valuable experience in learning what it feels like to telephone for help when you are not certain what you need. Keep track of how many times you are transferred, who offers to help, and who sounds interested in your problems.

17–4. Good behavior deserves to be rewarded. When you have finished, turn over the three cards and you will have some reminders of telephone practices that you can now use.

18

Employment Interview

For the time invested, the employment interview may be more important than any other communication in the dental office. A few minutes' conversation among strangers is the foundation for putting together a professional team and creating mutual expectations that constitute the standards for success.

Because the employment interview is so critical and abbreviated, there are guidelines for the type of information exchanged, interview timing, and location. The questions tend to be stereotyped and some are even prohibited by law. Extrapersonal communication—dress, handwriting, and use of time—must also be considered.

This chapter begins by defining the goal of a successful interview. A three-step process is proposed to show how questions appropriate to each stage lead logically to decisions that maximize the efficiency of hiring. We focus on questions that should be asked, inappropriate questions and how to answer them, and on communicating one's decisions politely but unambiguously. The process is considered simultaneously from the perspective of both the employee and the applicant.

GOAL: SEARCH FOR MUTUAL NEEDS

An interview is successful when it gives sufficient opportunity for dentists and applicants to discover whether employment will really satisfy both their needs over a reasonably long period of time. It is the testing and creating of a new work alliance. Dentists need employees who can perform important tasks quickly, effectively, and with minimum supervision; who are congenial and well-adjusted; and who can share an interest in the success of the practice. Employees have similar needs for compatible interpersonal relationships on the job. Additionally, most seek a living wage (as determined by their own expenses), opportunity to serve the public, a chance to learn new skills, rewarding interpersonal contacts, and status and recognition (represented by authority and pay above prevailing standards).[1,2]

But dentists, employees, and practices differ in the way they balance these and other personal needs. Interview communication skills determine whether a real, mutual fit in needs can be recognized. The worst case is where the dentist and the applicant either fail to understand their own needs or misrepresent them. This leads to surprises, disappointments, and eventually to termination or low-grade tension and poor morale.

THREE-STAGE INTERVIEW PROCESS

Figure 18–1 shows a model three-stage interview process. Preferences and needs may lead to some stages being protracted or combined, but keeping this structure in mind should facilitate interviewing communication. Different decisions are made at each stage, and these require different communication strategies.

In the first stage, contact is made and general compatibility is assessed (location and type of practice, qualifications of applicant). The second stage is devoted to exploring job requirements, policies such as salary and vacations, and the training and employment history of the applicant. The final stage is a detailed interview between the person ultimately responsible for hiring and the applicant. At each stage, a decision must be made by the employer and the potential employee. Either may decide not to continue to the next stage and must either ask to continue or politely end the process, with words such as those suggested in Figure 18–1.

Initial Contact

The employment interview begins at the moment the initial contact is made. This is typically done over the telephone and is an exchange of general information between the applicant and an office staff member.

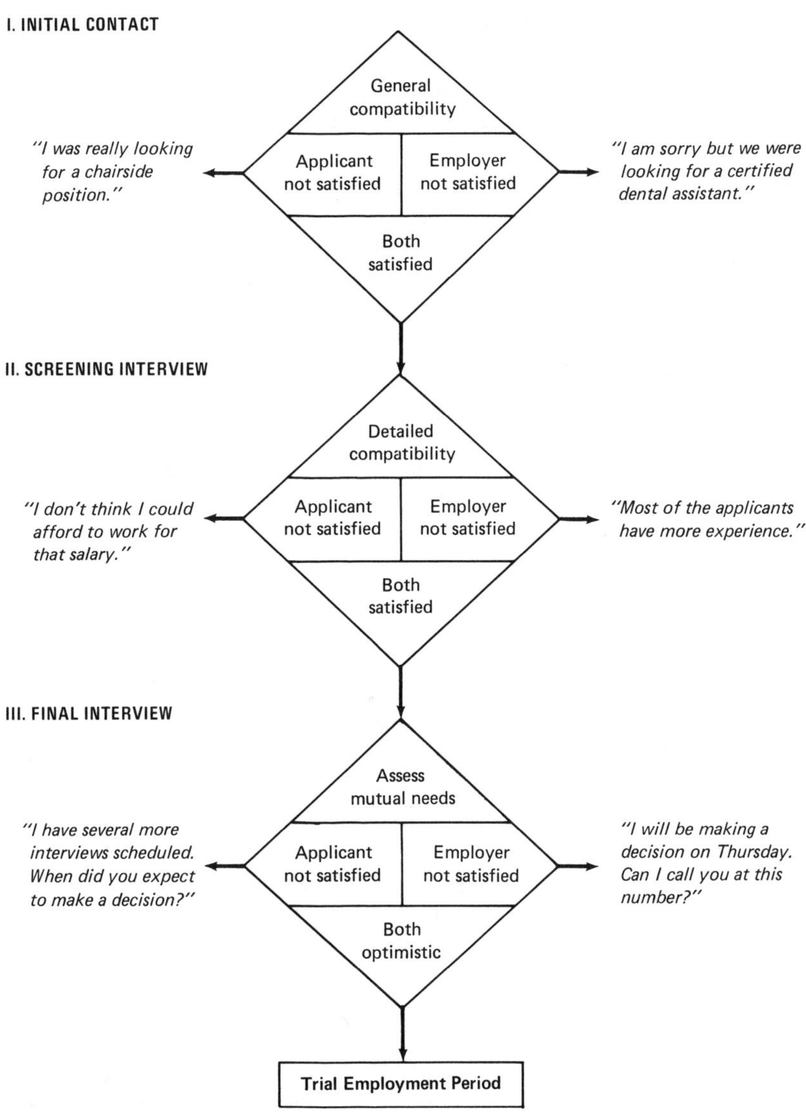

Figure 18–1. Stages of an employment interview.

First impressions are, minute for minute, more important than any other interaction.[3] Thus, they should be well prepared in advance. Both the applicant and the person responsible for screening calls should think through and write down the essential information and questions and have a pencil at hand to take notes. This creates a favorable image of being organized and efficient, and avoids the embarrassment of forgetting.

Figure 18–1 suggests what might be said if either party doubts that there will be a good job fit. If both parties wish to pursue an interview, the following information should be exchanged:

1. What should be brought: resumé, letters of recommendation, references?
2. When is the interview and how long is it expected to last?
3. Where is the office located, nearest cross street, where to park, which bus to take?
4. Who should the applicant ask to see?

Screening Interview

The purpose of the first visit to the office is to determine the applicant's general qualifications, to see whether the office appears to meet the applicant's needs, and to allow potential coworkers to meet each other. The screening takes place at the office and includes general and specific questions and a tour of the practice. The job description is reviewed and questions are answered about policy, salary ranges, other benefits, and other staff members. The office manual, which is where the job description is kept, should be reviewed. Educational and work background of the applicant are discussed. A tour of the office should include introductions to all staff who are present. A plain sheet of paper can be used to have the applicant write the following information: training, certification or licensure, work history and references (location, address, telephone, dates, and reason for leaving), and applicant's present address and telephone number. Except in cases of hiring associates or the initial auxiliary, office staff other than the dentist can conduct most of the initial screening.

The initial visit is characteristically informal. It is a time to explore expectations without pressure to reach a decision. The communication is social, conversational, and heavily weighted toward nonverbal, nonpersonal dimensions. Physical appearance and mannerisms are important in most working relationships.[4] The organization of the office, the pace, the patients, and the distribution of responsibility can only be communicated accurately by observation.

Effective use of time communicates personal control and consideration.[5] The applicant should be prompt and the staff should have set aside time to devote attention to the applicant. Job candidates have long been told to dress and groom themselves for an interview. This is still sound advice, but it should be remembered that clothes can lie. It should also be noted how the staff is dressed and how they relate to each other and to patients. The applicant's use of a plain piece of paper to record requested information, as opposed to professionally prepared resumés, communicates clarity of handwriting as well as ability to be complete and organized with minimal structure.

A *screening* interview should be used for exactly that purpose. Significant discrepancies between the employer's requirements and the applicant's talents should be sufficient grounds for terminating the interview at that point. If the job does not appear to satisfy the applicant's needs, it is not necessary to continue. All candidates who pass the screening and are scheduled for a final interview with the dentist must be acceptable to the practice.

Final Interview

Sometimes the pressures of time, characteristics of the practice, or personal preference make it difficult to separate the first visit from a distinct formal interview that leads to an employment decision. When it is possible to separate these two meetings, there are six advantages in doing so. First, by removing the pressure of having to reach a final decision, the initial visit becomes open to the informal communication that is a fundamental part of testing work alliances. Second, there is a large savings of time as only qualified applicants who feel comfortable with the office are allowed to proceed to an interview with the dentist or other ultimate decision maker. Third, this practice allows for a convenient scheduling of the final interview so as not to interfere with patient care. Next, it gives the dentist a chance to consult with the staff and to take their impressions into account prior to making a final decision. The fifth advantage is the time afforded to check references. Finally, it gives both applicant and employer a second chance to appraise each other. Any position worth accepting and any person worth hiring deserve a second look.

PRELIMINARIES. Prior to the final interview with each qualified applicant, the *dentist* should do four things: review applications, consult staff members who have met applicants, telephone references, and telephone applicants to arrange the interview. It is important that the dentist do this personally to learn first-hand how each applicant sounds on the telephone.

KEY QUESTIONS. The final interview should begin with some conversational remarks, followed by an explanation of the purpose of the second interview. Finally, an overview of the interview should be given.

- *(Dentist to applicant)* "I'm glad to see you again. I appreciate your coming back a second time. Paula and Kay were very impressed by you (conversation to establish rapport) . . . My goal for this meeting will be to give us both a chance to find out whether hiring you for the chairside job would be the best thing for both of us. You are clearly qualified and I'm not going to try to sell you on this office because if we aren't honest with each other now, we'll find out soon enough and that's no way to learn (purpose) . . . I have three or four questions that I would like to ask and then I'm sure there are some things I can answer for you (overview). . . .

The five questions that appear in Table 18–1 form the basic framework for an employment interview. There need be no hesitation about following small digressions as long as the central items in the interview are not obscured and each of the five points is considered for each applicant.

Applicant's Understanding of the Job. It is needless repetition for the dentist to describe the job—this should have been well understood by any applicant who has pursued the position this far. A recommended alternative is to ask that applicants paraphrase the job requirements, thus providing an opportunity to learn something about their communication skills. Gross distortions of the job description are symptomatic of significant unmet needs and a signal of danger. An accurate paraphrase demonstrates quick learning and promises a short training period.

Applicants should be prepared (and even rehearsed) to answer such a question, even if it is never asked. It is an excellent test to determine whether the position really meets the applicant's needs. It is also good preparation for the interview as a whole and helps identify questions that should be asked.

TABLE 18–1. PROBING KEY MUTUAL NEEDS IN THE FINAL INTERVIEW

What is Revealed in Question Answering	Key Questions	What is Revealed in Question Asking
Confirms realistic expectations, is a quick learner, good communicator and listener during screening interview	"In order to check our mutual understanding of this job, could you explain what you see as the most important duties of the job?"	Shows interest in effective communication, is not dogmatic, confirms accuracy of screening interview information
Relates job characteristics to personal needs, understands both	"Can you tell me what there is about this particular job that interests you?"	Cares about employee needs, wants employees to be satisifed
Can honestly appraise working conditions, demonstrates openness in answering difficult questions	"What was it you liked best/least about your last job? Why did you leave?"	Expects honesty and open communication
Shows familiarity with market, knows own worth, knowledge of job	"Based on what you have told me, I could start you at $650. Do you feel that would be satisfactory?"	Important factors are discussed up front, open to discussion
Shows interest in job, desire to assess potential for satisfying needs	"Well, I've been asking all the questions. There must be some things I can answer for you."	Is willing to initiate two-way communication. Openness, if answers appear candid

Realistic Personal Needs Assessment. A second question worth asking is "Why are you interested in this particular position?" Applicants who have only a vague response to this inquiry have not thought very deeply about the position, their own needs, and the match between them. What is being sought is an honest, accurate appraisal of the fit between the position and the applicant's talents and needs. Specific, concrete answers are preferable to generalities.

- *(Applicant to dentist)* "I am trained in four-handed dentistry and I have also taken some business courses. I think this position would give me a chance to use both because you really need some coverage at chairside and at the front desk as I understand it." (Good, specific response)
- *(Applicant to dentist)* "This is exactly the type of position I have been looking for and I really think I could do a good job for you." (Poor, vague response)

Realistic Assessment of the Office. It is useful to know how accurately an applicant has recognized the essential features in the office; it is also difficult to find this out. It may be useful to ask about previous employment experiences. "What did you like best (or least) when you worked in Dr. Singer's office?" This is one way of discovering what the applicant values in a work environment.

The response should be candid, specific, and not defensive. This is an opportunity for the applicant to express what is important and what is irritating about work. If the dentist agrees, there is a chance for a healthy, long-term job; if differences of opinion and values exist, it is better to have them in the open from the beginning. If a hygienist does not like working on a commission basis or working 30-minute appointments, this should be stated.

All applicants should be prepared to answer the question, "Can you tell me a little about why you left your last job?'

- *(Applicant to dentist)* "Dr. Bellinger's receptionist and I had some personal problems which were preventing me from treating patients with the respect I feel patients should have." (Good response, frank and specific)

If the dentist knows Dr. Bellinger's receptionist and finds him or her disagreeable, the applicant will appeal to the dentist. If the dentist admires Dr. Bellinger's receptionist, chances are excellent that this candidate would sooner or later come to grief over the same issues if hired. It should always be assumed that the dentist has checked references.

Salary and Working Conditions. Salary should be discussed during the final interview and the topic may be raised by either the dentist or the applicant.

- *(Assistant to dentist)* "The receptionist and I discussed a salary range of $700 to $750 per month. Now that you have heard about my training and experience, can I ask, if I were offered the position, what the salary would be?"

The applicant and the dentist should both be familiar with prevailing norms in the area but should not be reluctant to discuss modifying factors such as fringe benefits, special working conditions, experience, and training of the applicant. If the dentist and applicant can have a frank discussion about money at this point, chances are excellent that good staff communication will be possible if the applicant is hired.

Opportunity for Applicant's Questions. Finally, the interviewer should ask whether the applicant has any questions. Specific issues arising out of the screening interview or the conversation with the dentist should be brought up. If no other questions remain unanswered, it is appropriate to reflect the dentist's questions.

- *(Applicant to dentist)* "Does my understanding of the job come close to what you had in mind?'
- *(Applicant to dentist)* "Do you feel that I meet all of the requirements for the position?'

Answering, "No, I can't really think of anything just now" is a dull and uninspiring way to end an interview. Applicants should rehearse the closing question from the dentist and be prepared as the question is almost invariably asked.

INAPPROPRIATE QUESTIONS. Not every dentist is a skilled, effective interviewer even though he or she may be an excellent employer in other aspects. Applicants must be prepared for interviews under less than ideal circumstances. They should also be sensitive to the type of questions asked, as these will reveal something about the dentist's management style. Table 18–2 shows four inappropriate interview questions, what each may mean, and how to respond.

Control and Lack of Preparation. The first three questions in Table 18–2 reveal an interviewer who has some problems with objectivity.[6] The goal of the interview is to assess the compatibility of the applicant and the position. Instructing the potential employee, reading the application, or inviting comments with no structure may not achieve this goal; they certainly tend to waste time.

An effective response in each case is to respond politely to the question asked, but quickly refocus on the job and qualifications.

- *(Applicant to dentist who has been reading the resumé)* "Is my kind of background and work experience what you had in mind for this vacancy, Dr. McDowell?"
- *(Applicant to dentist who asked, "Well, what have you been*

TABLE 18–2. INAPPROPRIATE INTERVIEW QUESTIONS AND REMARKS

Question or Remark	What is Revealed About Interviewer	Appropriate Response
"I know you've heard this already, but I would like to review the job and some of my policies."	Control, authority, lack of trust in staff, fear of being misunderstood	(Listen, but at first opportunity) "Oh, then as I understand it. . . . (paraphrase) I do have a question though."
"Give me a few minutes to read this resumé. . . . Oh, I see you went to Carter college."	Unprepared, shies away from personal contact, tends to be formal, may be rushed or disorganized	(Wait, answer questions, but at first opportunity) "I think I really learned the most in Dr. Dooley's office. His practice is a lot like yours"
"Well, I don't have anything in particular. You just tell me about yourself."	Unstructured, may be defensive, and perhaps uninterested in people	"I trained at Jenson and worked in several practices . . . There are several reasons why this job seems very appropriate . . ."
"I noticed you just got married. Do you have any family plans?"	All such questions are designed to gain information felt useful for a better decision. Whether the question is discriminatory depends on whether it can be justified as job-related.	"I would be glad to tell you, but I am not certain how that would relate to my qualifications to do an excellent job?"

doing with yourself?") "I grew up in Chicago and after graduation I worked for a group practice for two years. I really enjoyed the challenge because the dentists were treating a lot of patients and the quality was high. But when I got married we moved and the commute is just unreasonable. Then I heard about this position. . . .")

Potentially Discriminatory Questions. Some questions in an interview may be offensive. Such items as ethnic origin, age, marital status, intentions of having a family, age of children at home, and personal health may irritate some applicants. If the questions are idle curiosity, the dentist is rude. If they stem from prejudice, the issue may involve job discrimination. In most cases, they are asked in a effort to learn information the dentist feels is important to filling the position.

The general rule is that all questions asked of applicants must be directly job-related. "Do you speak Spanish?" is relevant if a significant segment of the practice is Spanish speaking. If punctuality is important, then it is proper to ask how the applicant plans to get to work. If long-term continuity and regularity are vital (as in examiners for an epidemiological survey), then questions about health and family commitments are justified. In all such cases, it is prudent to state these requirements in writing as part of the job description and to explain the necessity for the questions prior to asking them.

Answering questions of a personal nature presents a difficult choice to some applicants. If a problem arises, it might be handled by responding in the following fashion.

- *(Applicant to dentist who has inquired about family plans)* "Of course my husband and I have discussed this but I'm not clear how that relates to the job."

The interviewer will either explain the intention of the question or apologize and withdraw it.

CONCLUSION. At the end of the interview, both the dentist and the applicant should state their feelings and should agree on what is to happen next. If the dentist feels that the applicant is qualified and would be an asset to the practice, this can be expressed. No job offer is implied by this remark because there may be other more qualified applicants. Applicants make an excellent impression by answering the final question with a reaffirmation of interest in the position.

The customary end of an employment interview is for the dentist to express satisfaction and appreciation for the meeting and state a date and time by which a decision will be reached.

- *(Dentist to applicant)* "Thank you for your time and interest in the job, Mary. I appreciate your candor. I expect to be making a decision by Thursday and my receptionist will call you regardless of what I decide. Is this number okay for Thursday evening?"

The employer and employee must independently decide from among three alternatives: (1) does not meet needs, (2) possibly meets needs but may not be the best available fit, and (3) exactly meets needs. A job interview ends in hiring an employee only when both dentist and applicant feel that no better alternative exists. Table 18–3 shows what dentists and applicants are likely to

TABLE 18–3. END-OF-INTERVIEW DECISIONS

Applicant (A)	Employer (E)		
	Applicant does not meet needs	Applicant possibly meets needs	Applicant exactly meets needs
Job does not meet needs	E: "I don't want to mislead you. The job we are filling requires someone with more experience."	E: "From what I see here you meet all of the qualifications. There are three other candidates. I will be deciding. . ."	E: "You really are what I have been looking for and I would love to have you start Monday."
	A: "I agree. This seems like a very high-powered practice."	A: "I really appreciate the chance you have given me for a thorough view of your practice. But I have some other interviews."	A: "I am very flattered by the job offer, but I really want to do some expanded duties."
Job possibly meets needs	E: "Several of the applicants are already certified."	E: "There are three more candidates."	E: "I think you could start . . ."
	A: "Yes, I was planning to take those CE courses at the University."	A: "I understand, I have an appointment on Thursday. But I really like this office. When will you make your decision?"	A: "Oh, that is great, but I promised Dr. Jenkins . . . I would like to see that office. How soon must you decide?"
Job exactly meets needs	E: "We were looking for someone with more experience."	E: "There are other candidates . . ."	E: "I think you could start . . ."
	A: "I really appreciate the chance to find out about your practice. After I get a little experience, there may be a position I could fill here?"	A: "I have an appointment on Tuesday. But of all the offices I have seen, this is the most impressive and I hope you will consider me when making your decision."	A: "I was hoping you were going to say that. This job really seems to meet my needs, too."

say in each of the nine possible combinations of personal assessment of the employment prospect. It should be noted that it is the person with the *least* interest, or the greatest unmet need, who determines the outcome.

CASE: REASONABLE ANSWERS TO UNREASONABLE QUESTIONS

Mable answered a classified advertisement in the local paper for a receptionist in Dr. Stockel's office. "Hello. My name is Mable Briggs," she said over the phone, "and I am inquiring about the advertised position as a receptionist in this office."

"Oh, yeah. I think that's still open," answered a harried voice. "I'm just temporary here. You'll have to talk to the Doctor and he's with a patient now."

"Very well. I'll leave my name and number. Is there anything you can tell me about the position?"

"No, I just started yesterday and I don't really know anything about it. Kinda hectic here, though. What did you say your name was?'

"I'm Mable Briggs, B-R-I-G-G-S. The number is 9-2-6-4-9-3-2 and I'll be here throughout the afternoon. If you could also tell me your name and when you think Dr. Stockel might call, it would be a great help."

The dentist called back that afternoon and after a brief chat about the duties and Mable Briggs's experience (an elementary school secretary for several years), an appointment was set for Saturday morning, a nonworking day in the office and at school.

That Saturday, the applicant found the dentist in the front office copying charges from a huge stack of charts. "Good," he said, "right on time. Did you ever see such a mess?"

"It looks like you could use some help."

The dentist dropped the chart in his hand and leaned back. "Let me tell you a little about how much help I can use." He talked for about ten minutes in a meditative way about how busy he was, how hard it was to get good help, and how the last front desk person had been so disorganized and then left with two days notice. He interwove his narrative with general comments about his own personality and what he expected from a receptionist: "I need efficient, organized people around me . . . everything must be quality . . . I want someone who makes my job easier, not harder." Finally, he leaned forward and said, "Well, if I haven't scared you away completely, why don't you tell me a little about yourself?"

"I am the part-time secretary at Sassarini School and I have worked there for four years, mostly doing attendance records, parent contact, and state reporting. You have a lot of paperwork, Dr. Stockel, but you should see what the state makes us do. My children are now all in high school and I'm looking for a full-time job, and for a challenge. Helping you organize your office would appear to be about the right size challenge, I would say. But there are many specific things such as hours I don't understand yet about the position . . ."

"Oh, right. There's lots more I haven't told you. For example, I'm looking for someone with insurance experience. I want someone in here as fast as possible. It's five days a week—Monday, Tuesday, Thursday, and Friday 8 to 5 and Wednesday 12 to 8. And the salary is negotiable."

"May I ask what range you had in mind?"

"Hummm, $650, $700 . . ."

"I think I meet your formal qualifications, Dr. Stockel, and what you have told me about the job sounds like it would fit with my experience. But I would love to see your office in operation. I am not working Tuesday or Thursday of next week and, if it's okay with you, I'd like to come in for a few hours to meet the rest of your staff and see the flow of paperwork. I'd even help a little if there is some simple filing or other jobs. I also imagine you'd like some time to review my resumé." She handed a copy to the dentist. "I tried to put down everything I thought you'd need to know, but I'm sure you'll have some questions. Mr. Pattersen, the Principal at Sassarini, knows that I am looking for a full-time position and he would be happy to receive a call."

"Well, Mrs. Briggs, you certainly seem to have it all together. And, sure, it would be fine if you came in on Tuesday or Thursday. In fact, I think that's a good idea."

"I'm glad," returned Mable, smiling and standing up. "I have really enjoyed talking with you. I'll be here Tuesday at one, and maybe we can talk again in detail after the last patient leaves."

"Okay, good," said the dentist, standing too.

ANALYSIS

In this case, the applicant has tactfully assumed responsibility for structuring the interview since the dentist did not do so. Notice for example how much specific information Mable was able to get from the temporary receptionist. She also correctly perceived that the office was not well organized and took the initiative to prepare a resumé and a list of questions. Mable also asked that the interview process be extended to include informal observation. It is likely that this impressed the dentist.

Mabel was tactful. She expressed responsibility and demonstrated organization. Review her speeches. They each began with a direct response to the question asked, no matter how inappropriate it might be. But then each response moved to focus on exploring mutual expectations and suggested a structure for the dentist. In every case, she had thought through the situation in advance and knew what should happen next.

The fact that the dentist is not an effective interviewer should not make Mabel less interested in the position. He may still be an excellent dentist and employer. But it is Mable's interpersonal skills and advanced preparation that will give them both an opportunity to find out whether they are in fact compatible.

REFERENCES

1. Morton, J.C., Clark, J., Adelson, R., & Hornsby, J.L. *Dental teamwork strategies: Interpersonal and organization approaches.* St Louis: C.V. Mosby, 1980.
2. Wiles, C.B., & Ryan, W.J. *Communication for dental auxiliaries.* Reston, Va.: Reston, 1982.
3. Jones, E.E., & Goethals, G.R. *Order effects in impression formation: Attribution context and the nature of the entity.* New York: General Learning Press, 1971.
4. Goffman, E. *The presentation of self in everyday life.* New York: Doubleday, 1959.
5. Knapp, M.L. *Nonverbal communication in human interaction* (2nd ed.). New York: Holt, Rinehart and Winston, 1978.
6. Bird, B. *Talking with patients* (2nd ed.). Philadelphia: J.P. Lippincott, 1973.

EXERCISES

18–1. With a partner, practice making responses to the following questions:

a. How old are you?
b. Are you married?
c. Do you have children at home?
d. Why did you leave your last job (or) why are you looking to change jobs now?

18–2. Make an inventory of the most and least satisfying characteristics for a job you now hold or the most recent one you held. Now list the questions you would like to have asked or the observations you could have made to determine these characteristics in advance.

18–3. Review the classified ads and select a position for inquiry. It need not be a dental position. From the advertisement, frame a list of questions you would want answered when you telephone to make the initial contact.

18–4. Review the case and assume that you are Dr. Stockel. Write out the questions you would ask Mable or role play the interview with a friend.

DISCUSSION OF EXERCISES

18–1. The first three questions may be discriminatory. The last one must be expected and an answer rehearsed. The sensitive questions may be answered if you wish and it is more important for you to know why the dentist is asking than for you to notify the interviewer that the question is out-of-bounds. For example, "I have two boys, 8 and 12. I imagine you're concerned that taking care of them won't become a problem for my job. Both of them go to their grandmother's after school and I think my references will bear out that this hasn't been a problem." In explaining why you left your last position, be honest. Expect that the reference will be checked. Also be fair to your last employer and emphasize the positive in what you are now looking for. "I had learned all I could in a general practice and I want more experience in surgery."

18–2. Many people find that the most important features of a job cannot be described formally or captured by specific questions. Often it is the way the questions are asked and the information given that provide the best clues. Third parties, references and other staff, are also valuable sources, as are direct observations.

18–3. Essential features of the position: nature of work, hours, salary range, location, starting date. Verify that you are qualified "on paper." Briefly describe your experience and training. Details of the selection procedure: process to be followed, key dates, interview time and location, what should be brought, who will the applicant be meeting?

18–4. Use Table 18–1 as your outline.

19

Speaking in Public

The type of interpersonal communication discussed in the first 17 chapters of this book cannot be avoided, but speaking in public can. Many dental professionals avoid public presentations because they see no reward or because they feel they do it badly. There have always been abundant opportunities to share knowledge with colleagues, participate in professional politics, and inform people about the benefits of dentistry. Ultimately, the image of the profession rests on the impression dental professionals can create in the public's mind. The ADA Strategic Plan, with its emphasis on marketing, stresses this opportunity.[1]

Whether the potential in public speaking can be realized depends on the professional's willingness to practice and learn the skills involved. This chapter provides a framework, a way of organizing and preparing to speak in public. Reviewing the suggested structure can hone the speaking skills of experts and can serve as a guide for novices. Everyone can learn to speak better in public, thus benefiting the profession, and derive satisfaction from such presentations.

Public speaking means one-way communication to a group of people about a preannounced topic at a prearranged time and place, and it is usually done by a person reputed to be an authority.

There are three sections in this chapter. The first deals with the context of the speech, showing how such questions as who will be there and who else is speaking can fundamentally shape the nature of the talk. The message, how it is organized and delivered, constitutes the second section. The final section involves the mechanics of public speaking: visuals, room arrangement, stage fright, and the other details that can aid or hinder a presentation. The chapter is written as a speech and each suggestion offered is illustrated by the text itself.

There is a single message that this chapter is designed to express: organizing a talk around the structure of context, message, and mechanics maximizes its chances of being successful. This can be summarized in the "rule of seven P's."

Proper
Prior
Planning
Prevents
Predictably
Poor
Performance

CONTEXT

Before accepting an invitation to speak, the dental professional should ask the 11 questions shown in Table 19–1. This may appear excessive before even agreeing to talk, but each question identifies

TABLE 19–1. THE CONTEXT OF A PRESENTATION: ELEVEN CRITICAL QUESTIONS

1. What?	The general topic your sponsor wants covered
2. Who?	The background, interests, orientation, and age of the audience
3. When?	Date and time of presentation
4. Where?	Location, general information such as city and specifics such as classroom, banquet, and so forth
5. How?	Format, formal speech, question and answer, panel
6. How many?	Size of audience
7. How long?	Overall time frame including questions and answers
8. What else?	What precedes and follows?
9. Who else?	With whom will the platform be shared, their views and assignments?
10. Purpose of meeting	In general, why is your audience there and what do they expect?
11. Action to be taken	What does your sponsor want to happen as a result of the talk; e.g., vote against denturists, brush and floss?

part of the context that controls the nature of what can effectively be said.[2] Sometimes the best speeches are those that are never made. If your sponsor wants you to teach school nurses how to brush and floss in 15 minutes, it would be better to decline, avoiding failure and embarrassment to both yourself and your sponsor. A "how to" course on nitrous oxide analgesia given to 150 persons in a lecture hall might also be wisely avoided. As the public has a tendency to view persons sharing a platform as peers, it may be well not to agree to appear with known cranks or people holding antagonistic views.

The questions about topic and audience obviously influence how one prepares for a speech.[3] The background and interests of the potential audience must be constantly kept in mind in organizing material, almost as though they were present asking "What did you choose that for? We need examples we can relate to. Don't go too fast." The audience also must match on other key questions, such as format and size. Formal speeches are deadly when the group is smaller than 30 persons.

The constraints of time, location, format, and duration must all be consistent with each other and with the purpose of the presentation. Meetings following dinner should be light in tone, short in duration, and audience participation (except for fun) generally should be avoided. Audience involvement, if desired, is greatly aided by a moderator. Long meetings need stretch breaks and these can easily be called by a speaker if overlooked by others.

Franklin Roosevelt had an unusual philosophy about the duration of his speeches. He used to say that it would take him a week to prepare a 5-minute presentation and a day to organize a 20-minute talk. But if something an hour or longer was wanted, he was ready anytime. In general, it seems to be true that short speeches are the most difficult to make effectively. Certainly the best remembered, such as the Gettysburg Address or Hamlet's soliloquy, are quite brief.

Each of the 11 questions in Table 19–1 identifies an element of the context that limits and controls what can be presented successfully. These limits may be so great or contrary that an invitation to speak should be rejected or changes suggested. But planning of the message and the mechanics of delivery should certainly be considered with the answers to these questions clearly in mind. The first step in preventing predictably poor performance is proper prior planning for the context in which the presentation is to be made.

MESSAGE

Each speech should convey one message, never more, no matter how long the presentation is. William James, the philosopher, physician, and founder of psychology in America, presented a series of lectures to educators that is available in the very readable book *Talks to Teachers*.[4] James advises that the limits of human memory and attention are such that no matter how long a person talks, the audience will attempt to summarize what is said into a single concept. A good speaker will do this work for his or her audience and will test the organization and cohesion of the talk against this rule: can the entire presentation be clearly summarized in a single sentence? If a member of the audience were asked by a colleague or spouse what you, the speaker, had to say, the listener should have a ready, short, and accurate answer.

To make it easy for the audience to identify and remember the essence of a presentation, two strategies are used: One involves the organization of material and the other is a matter of packaging or presentation.

Universal Outline Aids Retention

"Tell them what you're going to tell them, tell them, and then tell them what you told them." This cliché is the heart of every organized speech, as shown in Table 19–2. The message is presented three times: once in the overview which serves as a table of contents and permits listeners to organize what they are hearing; again in the main body of the talk where it is analyzed, explained, and illustrated; and finally in the summary where the key points are restated.

TABLE 19–2. UNIVERSAL OUTLINE FOR PUBLIC SPEAKING

Section	Purpose
Introduction ("Intro")	Build rapport, state general significance of presentation
Overview	State message, present preview of structure for presentation
Message	Present detail, examples, alternatives, conclusions
Summary	Restate message, review essential points
Conclusion ("Tag")	Engage the audience, point out their responsibility, call to action, thank them for their attention

INTRO AND TAG. The "intro" and the "tag" serve the special purpose of establishing a bond between the speaker and the audience. They communicate rapport.

Jokes, if one feels comfortable using humor and if they have a moral that can be tied to the message, are typically confined to the introduction. This is where the speaker puts the audience at ease and allows them to become familiar with his or her style, voice, cadence, and gestures, and where transitions from previous speakers and corrections of misleading introductions are made.

The conclusion or "tag" of a well-made speech goes beyond a summary of the main points. It "gives the speech to the audience." If the speech is persuasive in character, there should be a call to action. If it is informational, the audience should be reassured of the significance of what they have heard. An effort is made to give the audience a sense of ownership and responsibility for what they have heard, if by no other means than thanking them for their interest and attention.

Packaging Aids Retention

Lewis Carroll alerted us when he said, "It's a poor sort of memory that only works backwards." What a speaker must do to be understood is organize and highlight in advance to support the weak oral memories most audiences have. Ten ways of packaging a speech so that it can be remembered are shown in Table 19–3.

The following four memory aids function like "traffic signals" to guide an audience through a presentation:

TABLE 19–3. PACKAGING THE SPEECH TO HELP THE LISTENER

Structure	"First," "second," "finally," "the other major concern"
Signaling	"On the other hand," "in short," "even more importantly"
Nonverbal expression	Pace, pauses, inflection, volume
Illustrators	Pointing, gestures, return to podium before starting new thought
Repetition	Intentional redundancy of key points
Parallelism	Phrasing similar thoughts in a similar fashion
The "hook"	Catchy names for key ideas
"Ruleg"	State rules before giving examples
Anecdotes	Little stories as "breathers" in long talks
Quotes	Texture, variety, credibility

- The first such device consists of telling listeners how many points follow before making a major shift in topic.
- Another aid is to use conjunctions or phrases at the beginning of sentences that signal change in the direction of thought: "But," "contrary to what you might expect," "a fundamental exception," and so on.
- Similarly, nonverbal aids such as pace, pausing, stress, and inflection can direct listener's attention to important elements.
- Finally, illustrators and gestures that add emphasis improve the effectiveness of speech.

A college professor once lectured, using the blackboard only as a sort of tally card. Whenever he came to an important point he made a long mark on the board as if underlining a key sentence. Minor points warranted little ticks. At the end of the lecture the board was covered with a blizzard pattern of lines, dashes, and check marks. But each of us had good notes as we learned that he was using the blackboard to signal that we should listen, not watch.

Three more devices that make speeches more comprehensible are repetition, parallelism, and the "hook" A certain amount of redundancy is desirable. There is nothing wrong with repeating the essential message several times. The audience will remember what is repeated, not only because this aids memory but also because it is a clue to what the speaker regards as important. Similar thoughts should be expressed in similar language. The phrasing at the beginning of each parallel section of a talk should be the same and the phrasing that signals the conclusion of a section should be the same. For example, both the subsections on aiding audience comprehension in this chapter begin with a quote. Finally, the messages should be expressed, whenever possible, in a single word or phrase. Ad writers call such phrases "hooks," and fortunes are made with "we try harder" and "where's the beef?" Humorous hooks are especially durable. The hook in this chapter is the seven P's, which you will find repeated, in parallel form, at the end of each section.

It is good practice to introduce a general concept in a single sentence and then follow it with an example or two. This is the "ruleg" method of presenting material and studies have shown that this rule-first technique produces better learning.[5] It seems to work like the topic sentence that generally appears first in each new paragraph. The examples may be as short as the metaphor in the preceding sentence or as long as the personal anecdote about the professor who used the blackboard to underline visually what he was saying. Examples that connect with the experience of the audience seem to work best because they build rapport and because they shed new light on what the audience already knows.[3]

It is generally accepted and desirable to insert little stories or personal experiences in the context of long talks. An example is the oft-told story of the Harvard lecturer who pre-taped his lectures when he knew he would be in Washington consulting with the late President Kennedy. In this way, the teaching assistant could play the tape and the students would not have their class cancelled. On one occasion, just as he was leaving for the airport, the lecturer received a call that his business trip was postponed by several days and he decided to attend his own taped lecture. When he entered the outer hall of the auditorium he decided to listen for a while and critique his own delivery. He made notes concerning pace, monotony of inflection, need for more examples, and so forth. But in the end he concluded that this form of lecturing would still be effective because all of the essential ingredients of communication were there. He entered the hall to observe the effects of his taped talk on the students. What he saw in the front of the room was the teaching assistant sitting behind the tape recorder reading *Playboy* and, scattered throughout the hall, a handful of students asleep or with newspapers keeping watch over an enormous collection of recorders taping what was being broadcast.

All the ingredients are not present if the interaction between the speaker and the audience is omitted. As this story suggests, there is more to communication than the transfer of information.

This little vignette also illustrates five benefits resulting from the use of stories and examples. First, they communicate a point in concrete terms; second, they vary the pace and provide texture for a long talk; third, they are easy for the audience and presenter to remember; fourth, they are easy for the speaker to tell because the exact details are usually not important; and fifth, they can be omitted if time is pressing, or padded to fill a void. In short, anecdotes are small oases in a long talk.

Quotations can also be used to add richness to a presentation. As Christian Bovee put it, "Next to being witty yourself, the best thing is being able to quote another's wit."

Table 19–3 provides a summary of ten techniques for packaging speech to help an audience understand it. Together with the universal outline (introduction, overview, message, summary, and tag), they provide a general framework for effectively presenting a message to a large group when necessarily limited to one-way oral communication. They constitute the second step in preventing predictably poor performance through proper prior planning of the way the message is packaged.

MECHANICS

Once the context is known and the message is packaged, there still remains the final preparatory step of organizing the mechanics. This includes (1) provision for visuals, (2) prompts, (3) timing, (4) practice, (5) preview of the facilities, (6) attention to introductions, and (7) the nonverbal aspects of delivery (Table 19–4).

Stage Fright

Something should be said about stage fright. Amateur and professional performers alike experience it—only those who do not care are exempt. The difference is when the cold feet occur. Experiments with people learning to parachute confirm that as skill

TABLE 19–4. REHEARSING THE MECHANICS OF A PRESENTATION

	Type of Presentation		
Mechanics	***Formal***	***Semi-formal***	***Informal***
Visuals	Few, specially prepared	More, selected	Available and catalogued
Prompts	Written	Outline with key concepts	Note cards as references
Timing	Critical, plan 90% of limit	Know limits, plan anecdotes as fillers	Check with sponsor and audience during presentation
Practice	Read aloud	Review sequence and meaning of key words	Anticipate questions
Preview facilities	Check equipment and podium	Get away from podium if possible	Join group
Introductions	Add your own, verify accuracy of sponsor's data in advance	Add your own	Add your own
Nonverbals	Paraverbals and few gestures	Gestures effective, move about room	Same as for interpersonal communication

increases, the timing of fear moves forward in the performance of the act.[6] Novices report maximum anxiety during freefall. Pros are most nervous on the morning of the jump while still on the ground. The critical difference is that the beginner can do little during freefall to cope effectively with stress. The expert, while still on the ground, can consider wind, equipment, and personal health and alertness, and choose whether to jump or make necessary adjustments. Stage fright while giving a talk is debilitating. Apprehension in the preparation stages is normal and healthy. The authors have delivered addresses at national and international meetings and find that the maximum period of stress occurs after planning the message, just as preparations are being made for delivery. This is the critical point in proper prior planning.

Visuals

Visuals should generally be prepared after the message has been thought through and roughly packaged. This is especially true in dentistry, where the old saw applies that "an expert is someone from more than 30 miles away with a tray full of slides." There is a tendency for speakers to use their slides as a crutch, turning out the lights and talking about each slide in sequence. There are four problems here: (1) the existing collection of slides rather than the needs of the audience becomes the critical context, (2) the message is limited to the available slides, (3) poor technical quality can detract from what is being said, and (4) there is a danger of visual overload. If it is true that a picture is worth a thousand words, a typical carousel tray would be equivalent to 320 pages of text. This chapter contains only four visuals (tables), which are summaries of text roughly equivalent to a 30-minute presentation. Excellent graphic support can be developed to augment a well-designed message, but this typically entails a few slides of excellent quality. (The tables used in this chapter would make *poor* slides—they contain three to four times too many words.) Blackboards and overhead projectors are fine substitutes, where appropriate, because they involve an interaction of the speaker with the graphic material.

Prompts

For all but the shortest and most casual of presentations, some decision must be made about how the speaker will prompt himself or herself. Reading a typed (double spaced) speech is appropriate for large, formal presentations or where timing is critical, as in presenting research findings at professional meetings. Note cards should be used where the format is unpredictable but important since they can be rearranged or parts easily omitted. Appropriate situations include testimony at public hearings, debates, participation on a panel, or appearances before the media. Here, important statistics and quotes, together with their source if requested, should be written on 3 × 5 cards with a key word in the upper left-hand corner to facilitate quick access. Most cases fall in the less formal category that is covered by some kind of outline. The detail of the outline depends on the formality of the situation and the experience of the presenter. A good starting point would be to use the universal outline in Table 19–2 and add key words on the right-hand side for each point to be made or for each story or illustration to be used.

Timing

The more formal a speech situation, the more important it is to time it accurately. It is demoralizing to audience and presenter alike to be forced to make impromptu cuts at the critical point on a speech that is going too long. A good rule of thumb is to plan to talk only 90 percent of the time available. If the talk is well-presented, questions will certainly take up any slack time. When timing a formal speech, it should be read aloud, but in general a 10 page double-spaced typed paper requires 30 minutes to present. When planning an informal talk, there should be enough anecdotes and illustrations planned to control the length of the talk by skipping or stretching them as required.

Practice

It is important to rehearse any speech to give it a maximum chance of success. Formal speeches to be read are no exception. It is excellent practice to read them aloud several times so that the presenter can look away from the page frequently and long enough to maintain some eye contact with the audience. They may also be tape recorded and critically reviewed. Semi-formal talks should be rehearsed sufficiently to assure that all necessary key words are on the outline and that there is no confusion over what they mean. Informal presentations are best prepared for by imagining what the audience will be like and mentally responding to the type of questions they are apt to raise. In all cases, the first sentence of the introduction and the overview, and the first and last sentences of the conclusion memorized. These are critical points in a speech and not a convenient time for choosing one's words.

Facilities

The facilities should be previewed. It is a good practice to arrive early—early enough to mollify the fears of your sponsor that you might be late and early enough to adjust your talk or the physical surroundings if they are in conflict. Audiovisual equipment should be checked and the room rearranged if it does not suit your needs.

Introductions

Introductions are tricky and sometimes hazardous formalities. They are typically confined to establishing the credibility of the speaker, a fact that could probably be assumed by the audience's presence. They do serve a social function of transferring attention from the sponsor to the speaker, and short ones are usually most effective. Experienced speakers seem to prefer introducing themselves and often do tell the audience some of what they want them to know (usually of a personal nature), even following a formal introduction. There is wisdom in this practice, as it is part of the rapport-building process required at the beginning of a talk.

This point is illustrated by an experiment conducted at MIT some years ago.[7] A lecture was given by an unknown graduate student in a large social science course. His introduction was distributed in writing. It was five sentences long and existed in two forms—both were identical except that half of the class read, among other things, that friends considered him "rather cold," and half read that friends considered him "rather warm." Following the lecture, ratings by the class revealed that this single word in the introduction was critical. The audience primed for a "cold" lecturer reacted significantly more negatively. Observers recorded the number of questions and comments coming from students according to the introduction they had read. Students who had been introduced to a "warm" graduate student participated in discussion almost twice as much as students expecting a "cold" lecturer.

Nonverbal Communication

The way we talk and what we do while talking can add to or detract from the impact of a presentation. Of particular concern to novices are one's hands and the podium. For someone who worries about what their hands might be telling the audience, it is prudent to assign the hands some task. Holding chalk for the blackboard is preferable to fumbling with a microphone or note cards, even when the board is rarely used. If the formality of the situation requires a podium, the reading surface should be raised as close to eye level as possible with a few books to ensure eye contact, and the microphone should be properly positioned about six inches in front and four inches below the speaker's face before the talk begins. With smaller groups, the speaker should join the audience seated in a circle. An intermediary arrangement is to sit on the edge of a table or desk at the front of the room. This gives the appearance of openness with nothing in front of the speaker at the same time it provides wonderful support for nervous knees.

In a book on public speaking for women, Stone and Bachner[8] focus on avoiding the "self-defeating and self-trivializing" nonverbal aspects of communication that characterize the way some women speak. Chapters 4, 5, and 6 of this text also explain how this can be accomplished.

In 1964, psychologists in the continuing medical education program at UCLA presented a guest speaker on the topic of nutrition and fitness. Unbeknownst to the audience, this man, introduced as Dr. Fox, was an actor schooled briefly in the topic but essentially devoid of knowledge or experience. Because of his showmanship, however, Dr. Fox received strongly supportive reviews from the audience, who claimed to have learned a great deal from this expert. The "Dr. Fox Effect" has been researched enough now to support the conclusion that a smooth, professional, and authoritative delivery can aid substantially in communicating an effective message and can go a long way toward making up the deficit when the message is of questionable quality.[9]

Table 19–4 presents a summary of the seven mechanics of preparing to deliver a speech. They are a mental and sometimes verbal rehearsal of what is likely to be encountered when speaking. The value of rehearsing comes in keeping stage fright where it belongs, before the talk when something can be done about it. The third step in preventing predictably poor performance is to properly plan a rehearsal of the mechanics of the presentation.

SUMMARY

Despite the range of audiences, occasions, messages, and personal styles of speakers, there is a basic structure common to all of public speaking. It consists of probing the context (audience, location, time, topic, format, etc.) because a good speech out of context is ineffective and embarrassing. The message must also be packaged correctly because audiences need help in structuring what they hear. The universal outline and aids such as repetition, the "hook," and "ruleg" make what is said easier to remember. Finally, the talk must be previewed or rehearsed so that the mechanics of room arrangements, prompts, visuals, and timing, do not become distracting obstacles. All three steps are taken prior to speaking because proper prior planning is the essence of good public speaking.

Many people who find it easy to carry on extensive conversations or talk forever with friends and colleagues freeze at the thought of making a formal presentation. It often becomes even harder when they know they have something important to say. There is an intuitive sense that somehow the situation is different. This chapter explains what these differences are and how to handle them.

Speaking in public is a natural part of professional life, and like all skills it becomes easier and more rewarding with experience. We have suggested a structure and offered encouragement because we know the satisfaction that can come from a good public presentation.

The next response is yours.

CASE: PREACHING WHAT YOU PRACTICE

(This chapter may be read aloud as an example of a 30-minute, formal presentation without visuals designed for a mixed audience of dental professionals. For an analysis of the talk, see the exercises that follow.)

REFERENCES

1. American Dental Association: *Report of the American Dental Association's Special Committee on the Future of Dentistry: Issue papers on dental research, manpower, education, practice* and *public and professional concerns*. Chicago: American Dental Association, 1983.
2. Ehniger, D., Gronbeck, B.E., & Monroe, A.H. *Principles of speech communication* (9th ed.). Glenview, Ill.: Scott Foresman, 1984.
3. Taylor, A., Rosegrant, T., Meyer, A., and Samples, B.T. *Communicating* (3rd ed.). Englewood Cliffs, New Jersey: Prentice-Hall, 1983.
4. James, W. *Talks to teachers on psychology: And to students on some of life's ideals*. New York: W.W. Norton, 1959.
5. Evans, J.L., Homme, L.E., & Glaser, R. The ruleg system for the construction of programmed verbal learning sequences. *Journal of Educational Research*, 1962, 55, 513–518.
6. Fenz, W.D. Conflict and stress as related to physiological activation

and sensory, perceptual, and cognitive functioning. *Psychological Monographs*, 1964, 78.

7. Kelly, H.H. The warm-cold variable in first impressions of persons. *Journal of Personality*, 1950, 18, 431–439.
8. Stone, J. & Bachner, J. *Speaking up: A book for every woman who wants to speak effectively*. New York: McGraw Hill, 1977.
9. Naftulin, D., Ware, J.E., Jr., & Donnelly, F. The Doctor Fox lecture: A paradigm of educational seduction. *Journal of Medical Education*, 1973, 48, 630–635.

EXERCISES

19–1. Use Table 19–1 as an outline and determine the types of context where this chapter, considered as a speech, would be acceptable and where it would not. Some questions (3, 4, 8, and 9) do not seem to apply.

19–2. Use Table 19–2 as an outline and locate the sentence that begins each of the five sections in the universal outline.

19–3. Use Table 19–3 as an outline and review the section titled "Packaging Aids Retention." Locate examples of all ten packaging techniques.

DISCUSSION OF EXERCISES

19–1. (1) What: a general "how to" presentation of public speaking; (2) Who: dental health professionals of mixed background and experience with some assumption that they are familiar with the material covered in the first 18 chapters of this text; (5) How: formal speech; (6) How many: at least 30, preferably more persons in the audience; (7) How long: 30 minutes without questions and answers; (10) Purpose: assume interest in self-improvement and/or assignment as part of course work; (11) Action: audience should feel more confident in making a public presentation and have a structure to use systematically in preparing future talks. There are also a few "tricks" that can be borrowed.

19–2. "Intro:" page 273—Public speaking means . . .; Overview: page 273— There are three sections . . .; Message: page 274—Before accepting an invitation . . .; Summary: page 284—Despite the range of audiences . . .; "Tag:" page 285—Many people who find it easy. . . . The part of a speech that varies in length from a short to a long speech is the message. The other segments remain roughly constant in length.

19–3. (1) Structure: The first of four such devices . . .; (2) Signaling: Another way is to use conjunctions . . .; (3) Nonverbal expression: (when read, this paragraph should have a structured and balanced cadence that focuses on all four techniques equally); (4) Illustrators: (hand gestures, graphics, or blackboard use could mirror the pattern indicated by the block indented bullets); (5) Repetition: A certain amount of redundancy is desirable . . .; (6) Parallelism: (quotes at the beginning of the parallel subsections "Universal Outline Aids Retention" and "Packaging Aids Retention" and the seven P's); (7) The hook: Tag, seven P's, and the term hook itself; (8) "Ruleg:" (the paragraph that begins . . . It is a good rule to introduce . . .; (9) Anecdotes: (the story of the taped lecture); (10) Quotes: As Christian Bovee put it. . . .

Index